A389

THE COMPLETE
DIET BOOK

By the same authors

Cured to Death: The Effects of
    Prescription Drugs
The Long-life Heart
Hay Fever – No Need to Suffer
Persistent Fat and How to Lose It
Alternatives to Drugs
Immunity Plus

Arabella Melville, PhD
and
Colin Johnson

THE COMPLETE
DIET BOOK

GRAFTON BOOKS
A Division of the Collins Publishing Group

LONDON GLASGOW
TORONTO SYDNEY AUCKLAND

Grafton Books
A Division of the Collins Publishing Group
8 Grafton Street, London W1X 3LA

Published by Grafton Books 1989

British Library Cataloguing in Publication Data

Melville, Arabella
   The complete diet book.
   1. Physical fitness. Slimming. Diet
   I. Title II. Johnson, Colin
   613.2'5

ISBN 0-246-13182-9

Printed in Great Britain by
Hartnolls Ltd, Bodmin, Cornwall

Contents

Preface

There are two facts that every slimmer should know. First, people in affluent countries have been eating less, decade by decade, yet growing fatter. Second, more people diet every year, yet they also grow fatter.

This book explains why this is so. Part I analyses each leading diet and slimming system, and shows why the long-term failure of every new diet is not yours but that of the diet and the diet mentality. It tells you why your diet left you depressed, guilty and fat. Understanding the diet con will restore your self-confidence.

Part II solves the problems of slimming. Acknowledging that every person is different, it uses a series of questionnaires to pinpoint the individual action necessary for *you* to slim. The objective is to live in such a way that excess fat becomes a disadvantage to your body; when you do this you will achieve that enviable state of natural slimness.

In sum, this book explains how to live your life so as to become slim and healthy – for ever.

PART 1

Dieting be Damned!

CHAPTER 1

The Diet Con

Good news!

In America a revolutionary new diet treatment is proving almost totally successful for all those who use it. It only requires dieting for three days at a time! Now you can benefit from this new amazing breakthrough!

Nothing unusual so far, that is roughly the sort of thing you would expect to find at the beginning of this kind of book. You are probably a little suspicious, having heard such claims before and found they did not measure up in practice. Let us assure you in all sincerity, as serious writers and lecturers on health and related matters, that as far as we know *this* method really does work.

What is involved?

You go to a health spa. There you are put on a special slimming diet for only three days. As you would expect, advice is given on peripheral health matters, and you are generally pampered and encouraged. In such circumstances, with friendly people all after the same goal, who could fail? Very few; the success rate has baffled medical and slimming experts alike, many of the latter sadly refusing to accept the logic of this new system, despite incontrovertible evidence.

That is odd, because this highly successful new system is based completely on the accepted practices of slimming and diet experts. Calories are counted and closely monitored; participants are weighed regularly, and success rewarded. All the latest slimming foods are available. How is this method so successful when every unsuccessful dieter is familiar with all this? Success is based upon one crucial difference.

This system is used for people who want to *gain* weight!

Those who run the treatment centre are using a fact which many have observed: people who diet, although losing weight initially, generally end up fatter and heavier than when they started.

Dieting to becoming slim is like looking for the pot of gold at the end of the rainbow. When you set out, full of hope and enthusiasm, it seems a very good idea and you are sure you are making progress. But it quickly turns into an endurance test which soon becomes self-defeating. There is no pot of gold at the end of the rainbow. For most people there is no route to permanent slimness through dieting. It's a fairy story, a fantasy we create to give hope and make life seem manageable.

For 99 per cent of those who use them, diets and weight loss programmes fail. This means that for every hundred people who follow the trail of the diet fairy tale, only one will succeed. If these statistics applied to any other theory it would instantly be rejected.

For those who want a slim body that stays slim, reality may be harsh – that is, until you adjust to it. Then reality can offer far more than any fairy story.

Let's start with a brutal fact.

If you have bought a best-selling diet to try to shed fat permanently you have been conned.

The truth is that everyone who has tried slimming diets knows much more about failure than success. So you should not feel embarrassed; there are millions like you, quietly suffering because the latest wonder diet worked for a while, then left them worse off.

Neither should you feel guilty. You will discover, as you read on, that you were being encouraged to attempt the near impossible. And a cruel part of the diet con is that diet regimes are constructed so that *your* failure cannot be attributed to the diet.

This is not to say that people who devise best-selling diets are inherently wicked, although it may at times appear that way. As with all confidence tricks, the art of the successful con is to get people who are willing victims. This can make those who give bad advice and get rich from it seem worse than they may actually be.

Diets do not lack willing victims. It has been estimated that around 60 per cent of the adult female population (and a growing number of men) are either on a diet – or putting on weight between diets.

In this respect the diet market has the best sort of victims; not only willing, but prepared to come back for more, time and time again.

And the con works every time. Every new wonder diet holds out promises which remain unfulfilled. These range from the direct promise of 'shedding unwanted pounds' with miraculous ease, to creating a new vital and beautiful you with the implication that your lifestyle will become a cross between that of the Princess of Wales and Joan Collins – if only you stick to the diet, the whole diet and nothing but the diet.

At some level every dieter knows that the diet will not fulfil its promise. But as with all hopeless relationships, he or she hopes, against all the odds, against common sense, good advice and rational knowledge, that *this time* it will work. This time the transitory flush of success in the first few days or weeks will last, the slim butterfly will finally escape from the roly-poly caterpillar that ties it down, and by flying free all those secret yearnings will be realised, the heroine will marry the Prince, and live happily ever after . . .

Like all the best fairy stories, the dieting-makes-you-thin tale is just enough in touch with possibility to be accepted. The crumbling old castle where the action takes place is the idea that success is to be found in counting and controlling calories. This idea is not only built upon a false understanding of the way human bodies use food, but it also ignores the basic physiological functions of fat. This is enough to ensure its failure – yet *all* slimming diets are based on the same theory.

The diet con is based upon maintaining the erroneous belief that dieting will get you thin, that dieting must be based on restricted calorie input, and that this is the only way to be slim and beautiful. Yet the facts refute these beliefs. It is well documented that in Britain, for example, people are eating less and less every decade, but at the same time are weighing more. If low-calorie diets worked, after so many of them we would all be slim and sleek. Look around next time you go out, most people seem to be going the other way.

Why is this? One answer involves another part of the diet con. When you embark on a slimming diet, you are in effect trying a confidence trick on your body. You think you are saying 'Here is less food, please use up fat instead.' What your body hears is something different: 'Food is in short supply, prepare for famine and conserve fat.' Perhaps the question we should ask is: Who is conning whom in the tangle of conflicting interests provoked by slimming diets? You are trying to fool your body and it replies with a trick of its own; the result is, you lose. Meanwhile there appears to be no way out: everyone is trapped on a diet.

The reality is that dieting has become the religion of our age. Any appealing tale can be elevated to this status if enough people believe it to be true. The fairy tale becomes a myth and the myth part of belief; when enough people act on belief you have a religion. This is what has happened with the diet con over the past few decades. Diet books are collected like icons, many not read or followed, just possessed in the hope that they will exert a favourable influence. High priestesses deliver lessons through specialist magazines, some offering short-term diets to prepare you for that special date, a ritual cleansing common to all religions. Others discuss in great detail the latest products of the multi-million international diet industry. And everywhere millions take advice and follow diets purely as an act of faith, even though their past experience should cause them to doubt, question and reject.

For devotees of dieting religion this book will be sacrilege. We know that diets are a con, that dieting makes you fat. We also know that growing numbers of people are beginning to agree with us, and we hope to convince you as well.

When enough people can face the fact that they have been conned we will be able to tackle the problems of fat and weight control honestly and successfully. Although our approach in this chapter has been light-hearted, we are aware that being overweight is a very serious problem for many people. Do not lose heart, there are real answers to these problems for those who want them, as Part II of this book will demonstrate; meanwhile if you want to discover why your favourite diet let you down, find out about it in the following chapters.

When you have read this book you will be well on the road to successfully controlling your weight, fat and body shape – and that *is* a promise! You won't have a simple-minded diet to follow, and since you won't believe those fairy stories, you won't need one. After all, people don't go around looking for princes by kissing frogs, do they?

CHAPTER 2

Diets in a Nutshell

The elegant French have a phrase which sums it up very elegantly: *'Plus ça change, plus c'est la même chose.'* In the world of the popular diet, the more it changes, the more it turns out to be the same thing. The best-selling diet regimes that seem so different are in fact very similar. They make such a fuss about how new, how revolutionary, how unique they are for a very simple reason. They have to persuade people who have given up on the last diet that *this* new one is special. They want you to pay up in the belief that their formula will succeed where others have failed – that is the promise they all make to complete the sale.

We have analysed the best-selling diet books to discover their crucial elements. Here are the ingredients; you could write your own recipe and cook up a best-seller!

1. FOODS
Use a detailed calorie counter to work out a *low-calorie eating regime*. Don't be too fussy, it does not matter very much what foods you use, or in what order; your own unique mix will determine the flavour peculiar to your diet. Use your imagination, and remember, the more exotic the better! Just keep the average daily calorie count low, preferably around 1,000.

2. FAITH
The firm assertion that those who follow your regime correctly *will not feel hungry* must be repeated many times.

Add other supportive comments to reinforce this liturgy, such as 'few people in this country *ever* experience real hunger'. The object is to convince your reader that what she is feeling is not hunger at all.

3. AUTHORITY

You must be firm; emphasise that *discipline is good for you*. Bring out the masochism in your readers; this keeps them helpless, and makes your success easier.

4. LAPSES

Dieters have more than their fair share of human frailty, so you must anticipate lapses from the regime. Assert that *any* deviation from the diet, however small, will precipitate failure. Make sure that the blame for failure and the associated guilt is left firmly on the reader's plate, not on yours. You have to be subtle, of course; make it clear that any lapse will upset the cunning balance of nutrients/ enzymes/biochemistry or whatever you have laboured long to achieve on their behalf. This will cause the dieter to suffer dreadful consequences, like immediate fat deposition or irresistible hunger.

5. REASSURANCE

Emphasise the good; reassure your readers about the healthy nature of the diet. Cover yourself by use of the warning that everyone should always get their doctor's permission before starting on a diet – this can be done in a way that implies that your diet does not need this, but the sins of the less scrupulous force this cliché upon you.

6. THE GIMMICK

This is good for mystique and cover illustrations. Ideally your gimmick should be a particular food for which you can make miraculous claims, the miracle being revealed in the context of your clever diet! As in (1) any food will do,

but if it can be boosted with some pseudo-scientific properties, 'contains the rare and essential mineral/protein/
enzyme, etc', it is almost perfect.

7. PSEUDO-SCIENCE

An important tool in preparing your diet. Use it sparingly
to shade in doubtful areas or to add highlights where things
look flat. There is a lot of it about, but it goes off very
quickly, so you must take care to get it fresh and in the
right quantity; a hint is considered perfect. You will soon
learn how to handle it; the best source is your local library.

Mix the above ingredients together, serve with a light and
encouraging literary style, not too many long words or
difficult ideas, and be careful to keep the chapters short.
And *voilà*! Your success as a best-selling diet expert is almost
guaranteed. And if it does not work the first time, mix it
another way and serve it up again!

But what about the readers, the people desperate to lose
weight, to be thin, to be beautiful? Ah yes, you must not
forget them, for although the recipe may seem easy, if it
does not appear to answer *their* needs it will fall very flat.

Your diet must conform to the requirements of *the diet
mentality*. Over the past two or three decades the diet as a
way of life has come to be as much taken for granted as
detergents and double glazing. Many women know no
other way of eating; many mothers discuss the best age to
put their daughters on diets; all believe that dieting is the
only way to be thin.

That they are hopelessly wrong is irrelevant. The fact
that people in affluent societies are eating less every decade,
yet weighing more, leaves the majority unmoved. Even
detailed proofs of the hopelessness of dieting, such as
Geoffrey Cannon and Hetty Einzig's *Dieting Makes You Fat*
and Bob Schwartz's *Diets Don't Work* touch only the more
alert and receptive. Faith in the conventional calorie-
counting wisdom is undiminished despite the fact that

every dieter knows in her heart that it does not work in the long run. We should not be surprised; human history is littered with examples of majorities who got it wrong and would not let go.

Why do so many women believe there is no alternative to spending most of their lives on a diet? To find the answer we have to look at the case for dieting. It is based on very old-fashioned ideas about the way our metabolism uses food, and the function of fat on our bodies.

Calories are a measurement of heat. Food high in calories will produce more heat when burned than low-calorie food, as common sense will confirm if you compare a lump of meat fat with the same weight of lettuce. It is believed that if you eat more food calories than you use as energy, the surplus calories make fat. It is a very simple and attractive theory but like most such theories it is only partly true. In practice, it fails on many grounds. We all have metabolisms that are different, so different foods affect different people in different ways; the efficiency of individual metabolisms also varies widely. And we are not machines working to some dubious mathematical formula; living beings adapt and change and are subject to a range of influences, from the weather to our emotions. All of these affect our metabolism of food.

If this were not enough to sink the simple-minded belief in calorie counting, there is one factor which makes the nonsense clear. Crucially, fat on the human body is not just a store for surplus calories. For females fat is far from a passive store, it has four distinct functions. These are: to give sexual shaping after puberty; to act as insulation; to store surpluses; and to absorb toxins the metabolism cannot cope with. We will look at these functions in more detail later, for now it is important to understand that dieting, even if the idea were right, would only partly address *one* of these four functions.

Yet despite all the contrary evidence and experience, doctors and dietitians, food and formula manufacturers, all still subscribe to the validity of the calorie equation, so perhaps it is no surprise that the majority of people are encouraged to behave as if it were a basic truth.

Dieters want a simple answer. Like most people they do not wish to delve into the details of the problem; if they are getting fat, they want to know how to get thin. The calorie-controlled diet (eating less) seems to fit the bill, especially if some pseudo-science will imply that others have done the delving. Dieters will assume they are on the right track and if many others make the same assumption, they will all believe they are right.

If individuals fail to fulfil the slim promise of the diet, it then becomes *their* fault. They must have reverted to their bad old habits and eaten too much. Those who fail are left isolated with the guilt induced by the impossible task they have been set. The general belief in the possibility of success is never compared to the widespread reality. And it is a reality that goes beyond failure, for most dieters end up with more fat than if they had not bothered.

Of course diets do work, up to a point, and temporarily; but never enough to achieve permanent weight loss for the majority. The beauty of diets and diet books is that almost any diet will work just enough to maintain belief and hope. Those who stick rigorously to the regime will react to the combination of metabolic disruption and severe nutrient restriction by losing pounds. This is almost unavoidable when you subject your body to stress and deprive it of energy at the same time.

The diet is almost irrelevant: it is the *metabolic shock* which moves the weight. Any similar shock can have the same effect: love and/or lust, a strange environment, illness, bereavement or a sudden disruption in day-to-day life. The diet may only be useful as a focus of your motivation.

The problem is that humans are very adaptable. We recover from shocks fairly quickly. Our metabolism changes to allow us to continue as before, by adapting to what it interprets as famine conditions or shortages of particular foods, and our new foolproof diet does not work any more. No matter how virtuous, how firm your will or how much you suffer, you will eventually be beaten by the combination of adaptability and deprivation if you are one of the 99 per cent majority.

It is totally unnatural to try to live in this way, let alone to try to be slim and beautiful. If you are typical you will simply put the weight back on, but with more unshapely fat or flab which will be harder to shift next time you try out yet another diet. This is the diet seesaw; as your weight goes down and then up again your body has a higher proportion of fat to lean tissue. It is the method used by Bob Schwartz, author of *Diets Don't Work*, in the weight gain spas described in Chapter 1. He simply uses a three-day diet to set the seesaw in motion. Because your metabolism thinks it is living in conditions of cyclic famine, it does all it can to preserve as much fat as possible. It does this so that you will have a better chance of survival in a very natural reaction to your unnatural dieting.

As we shall see, many diet mixers have become aware of the calorie illusion and the problem of the diet seesaw. But they have not responded by changing to more effective slimming regimes; they prefer to continue as before, adding disguise to their products. The latest diet blurb will promise that you can 'shed unwanted fat without so much as counting a calorie!' The implication is that food is unrestricted; the reality is that the author has counted the calories for you. When you follow the diet you will get so few calories that counting is pointless. And indeed you can eat as much as you want, but you need to be as perverse as the regime you are following to top 1,000 calories a day by eating apples (or watermelon, or papaya or whatever) exclusively. Our appetite naturally switches off if we attempt to eat too much of any one food; the diet does not provide balanced nutrition and it sets off all the famine signals in our metabolism.

We estimated the average daily allowance in some of the best-selling diets that say you will not have to count calories. Most came out even lower than the relatively honest calorie-counting systems, and in general they produced a much worse nutritional balance.

The emphasis on self-discipline in best-selling diets is also unnatural, and it should not be necessary. After all, if the diet is going to make you feel (and look) fabulous, without a pang of hunger, why should you need to be so hard on yourself? If the diet is that good, it should be followed as a positive choice rather than because of negative denial. Starvation only feels good if you are very clever at deluding yourself about how you actually feel. Oppressive diets make a demand on the diet mentality; they require the dieter to add self-deception to self-discipline.

A high degree of motivation is necessary to change yourself into a slim person. Fat cannot be wished away, you have to be sufficiently determined to take appropriate action for long enough to persuade your body that it doesn't need all that bulk. But positive motivation is very different from self-discipline. Positive motivation produces self-reinforcement, whereby small success increases motivation, which in turn increases the degree of success. Imposed self-discipline immediately sets up conflict: you are fighting yourself and you cannot win. The battle usually ends in *obsession*. When this happens the diet mentality is complete; the victim is trapped and will suffer diet after diet, getting flabbier and fatter as she goes through life.

Where does self-discipline end and blinkered obsession begin? The diet that warns you will wreck everything merely by licking your fingers after making sandwiches for your family is obviously designed for hard-core obsessives. Other obsessive diets require you to eat only a very narrow range of foods, often just one or two in a day. It comes as no surprise that smart operators have developed packaged 'sole source' food substitute diets. Obsessive food behaviour requires you to shut out reality, for you might reawaken your suppressed desire for real food if you tasted a morsel of it.

Suppression of natural desire is just another battlefield in the destructive war dieters have with themselves. The twin forces of obsession and suppression lead to the creation of what amounts to food pornography. Every woman's magazine has its cookery feature, with loving, lingering close-ups of perfectly cooked full-colour food – food the average dieting reader would never touch. These articles are consumed in the same way that men consume pin-ups; the media treatment is similar, as is the underlying market mechanism. Both dieters and droolers would benefit from a little realistic involvement with the subject of their suppressed obsessions.

Food in this context is a source of anxiety. It has come to be seen in a light as unrealistic and impossible as the diets which have helped elevate it to this position. While the French get pleasure from food, the Germans much satisfaction and the Italians indulgent joy, Anglo-Saxons have turned it into a source of sin and guilt. Just as most of us cannot live totally free of sin, so most slimmers cannot hope to stick with extreme diets. Thus it pays to make diets impossible; it protects the diet and its guru by laying failure firmly at the sinner's door. You know failure is your fault, not that of the diet or indeed of the idea of diets in general.

This vicious flabby circle is tied together by amplifying the streak of masochism in all of us. Part of the female make-up is a tremendous capacity for persistence, it is a necessary part of the human survival repertoire. Women will put up with pain and discomfort that men would not consider. Within the diet mentality the guilt of failure is focussed on trying harder, suffering more hunger and deprivation, creating the belief that the more the dieter suffers the better (slimmer) they will be. It is a cruel illusion; they will only be better at suffering.

It may be simply a matter of mass fashion. Women have done more painful things than starve to the dictates of the

society in which they lived. Chinese women used to muti-
late their feet by painful binding over years; some African
women suffer clitoral circumcision and vaginal stitching
after giving very painful birth; in our grandmother's time
some women had ribs broken or surgically removed to
produce slim waists. Today all of this seems barbaric and
horrible. Will our self-inflicted metabolic mutilation seem
just as unbelievable to our grandchildren?

It is one of the strangest paradoxes of our time that
people who are voluntarily suffering starvation in one part
of the world are moved by the plight of others for whom it
is the normal state. It is even stranger that, although the
volunteers understand that starvation ruins health by damaging vital parts of the body, they continue to deprive
themselves. The results are predictable: dieters are listless,
lacking in vitality and energy; they suffer a variety of
metabolic disorders; they are more prone to infections and
they are laying a firm foundation for ill health as they get
older. This is what happens to all malnourished populations, whether volunteers in their own destruction or not.

Suffering reaches its height with the sacrificial virgins of
the dieting world, the anorexics. Their brittle, fragile fading
is hypnotically admired and feared. It is seen as a supreme
expression of faith in the diet ethic, combining obsession,
self-discipline and total denial of reality. Some diet writers
hover on the fringe of anorexia, displaying many of its
psychological features. Is it healthy, or even sane, to see
your bathroom scales as your lover? Or to have your life
dominated by the arbitrary arithmetic of how many pounds
you deviate from some handed-down ideal? The kindest
way to view such obsessions is in exactly the same way as
anorexia, as signs of deep emotional disturbance.

Here we find another self-sustaining circle. Emotional
disturbance can be both a cause and a consequence of
obsessive dieting. The nutritional deficiencies endured by
long-term dieters, combined with the physical and emotional anguish, will in time produce nervous tension,

insomnia and depression; the mind suffers as the body is punished. There are diet regimes which might be designed to increase neuroticism, and presumably the neurotic victims see their salvation in the next diet. They are hooked, and more of the same will keep them hooked.

Once you believe that dieting is the way to be thin you are likely to be led into the diet trap. The seesaw of weight loss and fat gain will be set in motion and it will be difficult to get off. Tragically, mothers who fail on perpetual diets lead their daughters onto the same fruitless path; thus the cultural myth that the only way to be thin is to diet is perpetuated.

The truth is that *none* of the best-selling diets we look at in the following chapters, whatever its marginal virtues, offers an effective long-term means of fat reduction or weight control.

You will lose pounds of body weight when you start any diet, but either your metabolism will adjust or you will not be able to live on the regime. The result will be weight and fat gain; it is unavoidable.

For slimmers, when weight loss is rapid the subsequent gain is also very fast. This is usually because the principal effect of the initial metabolic shock is to cause water loss from the body. Rapid loss happens fastest with low-carbohydrate, high-protein diets (such as the Scarsdale Diet, Chapter 4) and very-low-calorie formula diets (such as the Cambridge Diet, Chapter 3). The body quickly recovers its fluid content; these diets are characterised by diminishing returns.

Diets that include a higher proportion of carbohydrate do not produce such rapid water loss. Indeed, if you have been living on highly refined processed foods, changing to a high fibre diet (such as the F-Plan Diet, Chapter 6) will cause your intestine to hold more water, so the overall effect will be less dramatic. Basically, you are just moving water from one part of the body to another.

The ultimate test of any diet is this: does it really persuade your body to shed fat? The usual answer is that it does not. Dieters lose a high proportion of healthy lean tissue with any fat that they may shed. Lean tissues are muscles and the vital organs of the body, the body's protein content. Some vital organs are also muscles, the heart for example, and losing tissue from these organs is potentially very dangerous.

To counter these acknowledged dangers some diets include a high proportion of protein. The claim is that these diets spare the body's protein stores and cause you to burn fat selectively. This is a good example of pseudo-science; it is also pure nonsense! Any low calorie regime will cause your body to use up lean tissue. The fat will persist and your muscles melt away. Your body will react to starvation by *conserving* fat stores. This is logical in nature's scheme of things; as well as suffering famine, you might be pregnant or about to conceive. If you were, nature would consider it better for the baby to survive, so fat will be stored against that chance.

This response is heightened in our culture. The combination of voluntary starvation, a sedentary lifestyle and relatively high rates of sexual stimulation, mean that the conservation of fat is bound to take priority. In these circumstances, the metabolism will judge muscles and other lean tissues to be less important. Yet it is healthy muscles and well tuned organs that give the desirable shape and vitality that dieters so desperately envy in others!

Those who tend not to use their bodies, who do not enjoy physical prowess, who have not developed a deep sensuality of being, will tend to shed muscle more than others. Many of us, brought up with a lack of appreciation of our physical selves, find it easy to reject all our fleshiness without discrimination. The diet mentality reinforces the sinful view of flesh; for some dieters the self-deprivation and denial are based on the self-destructive view that all flesh is bad flesh . . .

It is time for our disclaimer. Of course slimmers, as

individuals, will show a wide range of individual variability in their response to dieting. A very small number can be slim and happy, if not healthy, on a diet. There will also be some who are so badly affected by a particular regime that it proves fatal. We are primarily concerned with the dieters in between these extremes: those whose desire is desperate, whose efforts are sincere; those who are misled, and end up with more fat than they started with; those who are the typical victims of the diet mentality.

The final flaw in all diets is that they do not take account of individual variability. Their creators produce a blanket regime, assuming everyone is exactly the same, that our lives are as predictable as those of battery hens, and that our food and nutrient needs are identical. Every time you see a diet with a week's menu as a precise step on the promised path to salvation, you will know that it was never designed to fit you.

In reality we each need a diet that suits our changing individual needs. Ideally we will choose to eat what we need, with confidence that our choice is right for us. We will take account of all the factors in our lives, and relate food to pleasure and nutritional fulfilment. We will understand that food, physical activity and emotional state are all part of a live interactive whole. No simple-minded diet can have the influence claimed for it on our lives or weight.

In a nutshell, diets make money – they do not make people thin.

CHAPTER 3

Very-low-calorie Diets

There are fashions in slimming, just as in every other aspect of modern life. The very-low-calorie diet (VLCD) is today's method. It is the ultimate in convenience dieting using a carefully formulated substitute for food.

VLCDs represent the high-tech solution to weight problems, sold with an elaborate façade of academic and scientific respectability. The most famous and widely used is the Cambridge Diet, developed by the biochemist Alan Howard. It was intended to be 'the perfect diet' and is sold as though it were just that. As we write this book, the promotional literature maintains that the Cambridge Diet is 'a complete balanced diet' and that it 'contains all the nutrients, vitamins and trace elements you need in just 330 calories a day'. However, Cambridge Nutrition have informed us that, in response to recommendations made by government experts, there would be a new formulation from 1 August 1988 which would contain slightly more fat and protein, providing 400 calories a day for women and 500 calories for tall women and men.

Other diets based on the same principles have been developed and are, in the main, minor variations on the same theme. Some contend that they are superior: a Micro Diet sales lady told us her product contained more protein (though what it might have had *less* of, she did not know); the Swift Diet is higher in fibre; but none is more successful than the Cambridge in financial terms. Cambridge Nutrition's turnover in 1987 was £7 million and the empire continues to expand rapidly.

It is easy to understand the appeal of VLCDs. All the dieter needs to do is buy a total food supply for the weeks ahead from a single salesperson. This person is also the diet counsellor, offering advice and support to her clients. Three times a day, the meal is the same: a concoction of nutrients made up into an instant drink with water. It is popularly called 'going on the soups'. Those who want something to chew can vary the diet with meal bars which may be used instead of the drink. Dieters are advised to take at least three additional pints of water each day, but no other food is allowed.

At this level of energy intake, people lose weight as fast as though they were taking in no food whatever. In many ways, the body reacts as if it were starving. Taking a VLCD does not significantly alter the sensation of starvation; it just makes it a less worrying process. You are unlikely to go blind on a VLCD, and less likely to die than if you simply starve.

For the dieter, contact with food can be severed completely. She doesn't have to consider the question of what she should eat. All she gets is her starvation supplement. In fact, it is a regime so close to starvation that the body produces a starvation reaction which can suit the dieter's purpose very well.

The starvation reaction is useful because starving people lose their appetites after about three days. Hunger may not return until they get a bite of real food. Meanwhile, they feel light-headed, with unusual nervous energy. It is a response which allows humans to function during periods of famine, so that they can do whatever is necessary to survive. The sensation will be familiar to anyone who has fasted for more than a couple of days.

If a slimmer can endure the first three days on a VLCD (and the counsellor is trained to help her through this difficult period), she can expect rapid weight loss with negligible hunger. As she starves, so she loses weight.

Everyone loses weight on 500 calories or less a day. Many people lose weight very quickly.

No wonder 'the soups' are so popular!

After four weeks, dieters are supposed to cease their strict adherence to the VLCD and eat one calorie-controlled meal each day for a week in addition to their basic drinks or bars; then they can return to four weeks on the VLCD as the sole source of nutrition. This sequence can continue indefinitely. Surveys have shown that, in fact, few users bother about the week with the extra meals, for it slows down weight loss and, paradoxically, induces a sensation of desperate hunger. So many continue on the VLCD alone for months together.

This system is sold like a medicine to doctors. But just as there are no medicines without side-effects, so there is no magical answer to a weight problem. The body reacts to starvation in several ways at once, and many of these are far from convenient or desirable. Those unwanted reactions should not be ignored. They are an indication of the inherent dangers of VLCDs.

Some people get early warnings of VLCD hazards; they feel ill from the start. We have heard from many people who vomited and suffered intestinal problems on the Cambridge Diet. Sadly, so determined were some of these women to lose weight (as promised in all those ads), that they continued to live on a diet to which their stomachs reacted as if to poison.

Marjorie described how her husband was so horrified at her state after four days on the Cambridge Diet that he called the doctor. She was 'vomiting white stuff, and kept passing out'. To the doctor the pattern of symptoms must have been very familiar, for he immediately asked where she kept her diet. When Marjorie discovered that her doctor had thrown her supply in the bin, she bought more for another attempt. This time her effort landed her in hospital. It was a new experience for her to be nursed without sympathy, having brought illness upon herself.

Reports in scientific journals and the experience of many dieters confirm that VLCD users endure a high incidence of unpleasant side-effects. These include persistent headaches, nausea, constipation, colonic spasm, cold intolerance, skin problems, hair loss, brittle nails, blackouts, dizziness and a furred, leathery tongue. Those who live and work with VLCD users have to put up with someone who is tired, inefficient and irritable, and whose breath stinks.

These are all symptoms of starvation. Starvation is not just a passive melting-away of the body but a disturbed metabolic state. Starvation – with or without a VLCD – causes sleeplessness, agitation and exhaustion. Sustained physical activity becomes impossible as the body consumes itself to keep the dieter alive.

The balance of nutrients in the VLCD was designed to allow theoretical survival for long periods. This was an attempt to create 'a perfect food'. It is a concept born of the astonishing arrogance of scientists who imagine that they know enough about human nutritional requirements to be able to create a synthetic food substitute. The fairy-tale castle has metamorphosed, turning into a fantastic high-tech laboratory where scientists attempt miracles.

Of course, the reality is different. VLCDs are not nutritionally complete. With each year, another nutrient is discovered to be essential to human health; such newly discovered vital dietary components will be missing from the current generation of VLCDs. How can the manufacturers hope to include the vitamins and trace nutrients that may not be recognised as necessary until next year, next decade?

The consequences of such omissions can be serious. Recently, a group of scientists at the US Government's Human Nutrition Research Center in North Dakota observed that the mineral boron is essential to hormone balance in women. Boron deficiency leads to oestrogen deficiency (cause of the unpleasant symptoms of menopause) and to softening of the bones – osteoporosis – in elderly women. The Cambridge Diet does not include boron in its list of minerals. Nobody knows how many broken bones can be attributed to its use; this is just one of many questions that the doctors and scientists who reassure us of its safety have not thought to ask.

No doubt the manufacturers of VLCDs will endeavour to include each new essential nutrient. But since doctors and scientists constantly discover more of the tremendous range of natural substances that keep us healthy, claims that any synthetic product is nutritionally complete cannot be valid.

Scientists do not know how many nutrients are essential, and they do not know how much every person needs of each. The methods by which our needs are assessed are imprecise, and to complicate matters, individuals vary tremendously in their needs. To remain healthy, you may need ten times more of a particular nutrient than your neighbour, and ten times less of another.

While our requirements for most nutrients may be close to average, we are all likely to need some nutrients in unusually large quantities. And although we are very unlikely to know what these particular nutrients may be, while we can select our own diet from a range of natural foods, our appetites will guide us. Subsisting on a VLCD formula does not allow any selection according to individual need.

The concept of the VLCD is based on the erroneous assumption that everybody is the same; that we all have the same needs and that the same quantity of a nutrient will suffice for everyone. In the short term, this may work well enough for previously well-fed people who have good stores of nutrients in their bodies, but in the long term, deficiency of an element like boron could make the crucial difference between a fall causing a broken hip or just a bruise. Because there is wide individual variation, VLCDs will produce individual nutritional imbalances which could cause all sorts of long term health problems.

The following factors are known to affect nutrient requirements:

1. The physiological state of the individual. This varies from time to time, depending on activity level, work load, emotional state and status in life.

2. Body size, sex and age.

3. Physical activity. This may be less of a problem with VLCDs than under normal circumstances – because sustained physical activity is so difficult under conditions of near-starvation.

4. Changes in the weather.

5. Medication use.

6. Illness and injury.

7. Previous availability of nutrients.

In view of all these factors, it makes no sense to put anybody on a standard diet – let alone suggest that a formula diet meets everyone's nutritional needs!

The assumption that we know all about human nutrition can cost lives. Looking back in our history we can see occasions when such assumptions caused deaths. Remember the sailors who died by the thousand from scurvy – deficiency of vitamin C – because ships' masters assumed that fruit was not essential to health? And Scott, who might have survived the Antarctic if vitamin-rich foods had been chosen for his expedition?

Early versions of VLCDs (also known as liquid-protein diets) caused sixty reported deaths in America, but because of faults in reporting systems, we can be sure that many times this number went unrecorded. Dieters suffered fatal disturbances of heart rhythm. The problem with these early VLCDs was said to be caused by their poor nutritional balance, but this has not been proved. We believe that long-term starvation *in itself*, with or without a VLCD, is dangerous to health. Heart problems are a particular risk. (These and other dangers are discussed further in Chapter 4.)

Extreme food restriction produces a unique combination

of hazards which cannot be overcome simply by adding extra protein or minerals to a starvation supplement. Lack of knowledge or understanding of the underlying problems mean that the manufacturers' simplistic attempts to render starvation safe must continue to fail.

The problem with fast weight loss through this sort of diet is that lean tissue is lost from the body, and especially from the heart muscle. This happens even when the diet contains as much high-quality protein as the body can use, because lean tissue cannot be conserved if the diet contains insufficient *carbohydrate*. At the same time, minerals, particularly potassium, calcium and magnesium, are lost from the body *even when they are included in the VLCD formula*. Research on the effects of VLCDs has revealed that adding these minerals to protect the heart has negligible effect.

To add to these hazards, quick weight loss causes release of a range of potentially hazardous substances from rapidly diminishing fat stores. To quote a standard medical textbook, *Toxicology: The Basic Science of Poisons*, there will be 'a sudden increase in concentration of chemicals in the blood should there occur a rapid mobilization of body fat'. According to the authors, Drs Casarett and Doull, 'storage depots' – in other words, that unwanted fat – 'should therefore be considered as protective organs'.

The health danger represented by the sudden release of chemicals stored in body fat will vary greatly between individuals. Some people, particularly men, will be able to cope; but there are others who, because of medication use, liver damage or diminution of de-toxifying capacity through long-term dieting, will not be able to metabolise these substances at the rate at which they are released into the bloodstream. They will soon begin to feel very unwell. Effectively, they are being poisoned.

In many clinical studies of VLCDs, between *one-third and a half of all participants drop out* and their experiences may not be reported. These people, although sufficiently motivated to enrol in the research, find the side-effects of living on the VLCD intolerable. Such a high drop-out rate means that the results of these studies are unreliable. The participants have been selected: they are those who can stand the regime.

A scientific image is crucial to the marketing strategy of the Cambridge Diet. To maintain it, research papers which can be used to extol its safety and effectiveness are essential. These form the material that allows the idea to be sold to doctors who in turn recommend it to their patients. Many such papers have been published, but we are not persuaded that the apparent benefits reported are valid for most dieters who might consider using the method.

While the research may seem convincing, the British Medical Association's Board of Science was sceptical. Concerned at Cambridge Nutrition's efforts to sell through family doctors, the BMA spent months investigating VLCDs and concluded that they could endanger health. They warned doctors that they might be held legally responsible for their patients' illness if they supported their use.

In a radio interview after concluding the investigation, the BMA spokesman, Dr John Dawson, gave a public warning. 'You can't go on on this sort of thing for ever. So we're concerned that first of all you lose protein; when you stop using the diet, you tend to put weight back on; in doing so, you tend to put back on fat, rather than the protein you've lost. Some people use these diets more than once and may get more protein loss the second time and will then put back weight when they stop using it, and they put back the fat, not the protein. At the end of the day you have to try to change your eating habits . . .

'If you lose protein and don't replace it, and if you then go back on the diet again, then there are possibilities that you could lose protein to the extent that might be dangerous.'

Much of the scientific support for the use of VLCDs comes from papers published in the *International Journal of Obesity*. This journal was founded and edited by Dr Howard, the man who developed the Cambridge Diet. We believe that there is bound to be bias in the selection of papers for such a journal – but most readers will not be aware of this.

Independent scientists have been critical of research reports on VLCDs. In some papers, only the lowest weights achieved by the individuals who did best on the diet are quoted, thus inflating the apparent size of the losses achieved. The reported rates of adverse effects tend to be lower than the drop-out rates suggest. In addition, most studies include only grossly overweight people – those still-rare individuals who are twice the normal weight for their height, or more. They will suffer far less on a VLCD than a chronic dieter with a stubborn stone to lose.

For these and other reasons, many nutritionists believe that the research fails to confirm the safety of VLCDs. In the United States, the Government Food and Drug Administration has insisted that the 330 calories a day formula is inadequate. The British DHSS Working Group on the use of very-low-calorie diets in obesity was also critical. Their conclusions were that women should not have less than 400 calories daily, while men need over 500; and they recommend that people who are only slightly overweight should not use them at all. Specifically, people with a Body Mass Index – calculated as weight (kilograms) over height (metres) squared – over 25, should not use these products. One after another, governments are demanding that the original concept of the VLCD be modified because the risk to users is unacceptably high.

There is a second persuasive reason for avoiding VLCDs which has nothing to do with controversy about their safety. This is their lack of long-term effectiveness.

The metabolic rate of people who use VLCDs declines so profoundly that many find that the pounds pile back on staggeringly fast on even the sparsest of real food. And while the weight they lost came from a mixture of fat and lean tissue, the pounds they regain after the diet contain a much higher proportion of fat. The long-term outcome is that the dieter gets steadily fatter as her weight seesaws. As she grows fatter, her metabolic rate falls and progressively smaller quantities of food are needed to make her fatter still.

As the cycle continues over months and years, the dieter's body composition changes. Studies of starvation have shown that some lean tissue is *never* replaced – except by fat. So the dieter grows fatter and fatter. Even when her weight is low, she will look like a blob because she has lost the lean tissue which gives the body shape. According to Dr John Garrow, Professor of Human Nutrition at St Bartholomew's Hospital Medical College, 'Some survivors of prison camps never regained a normal lean body mass and patients recovering from anorexia frequently have a struggle to avoid obesity because of low lean body mass and hence a low metabolic rate . . . A very rapid weight loss should not be seen as a benefit, but as a warning that lean tissue is being unnecessarily sacrificed.' He therefore believes that VLCDs are not an appropriate treatment for obesity, and unsuitable for casual use in slimming.

We should not leave the subject of VLCDs without acknowledging that some people feel well on them, sometimes markedly better than when eating their normal food. Arthritis sufferers can recover on VLCDs; some multiple sclerosis sufferers are now using them in the belief that their symptoms are relieved. Do they then have a value as therapeutic diets?

The VLCD formula can be better for its users than their normal food – if they habitually eat over-processed, nutrient-poor, chemically contaminated and unbalanced products typical of the diet of affluent countries. For previously malnourished people, the nutrients in the VLCD could work wonders. But this is an indictment of the dietary habits of these individuals, *not* a valid reason for using a VLCD.

People who are allergic to components of their normal diet may thrive on a VLCD if it does not contain the

substances to which they are sensitive. In these circumstances, absorption of the nutrients they need will also be
improved on the VLCD. So the condition of people who are
sensitive to common foods can improve on a VLCD, just as
it will on the elimination diets used in allergy clinics.
Arthritis is one condition which is quite often related to
food allergy, and those who find that they are free from
aches and pains when they use a VLCD as the sole source
of nutrition should try to find out which components of
their normal diet produce their symptoms.

Food allergy sufferers should not assume, however, that
a VLCD is the answer for them. Some contain synthetic
additives which can precipitate allergic reactions. Most
contain milk and soya protein, both common allergy triggers. Depending on a VLCD will make allergy problems
much worse for those whose symptoms are triggered by
components of the diet.

Whether VLCDs help with multiple sclerosis is still a
controversial question. It seems that some patients do
better, some are unaffected. There is accumulating evidence
that MS is affected by dietary habits and is probably linked
with reactions to toxic substances in the body to which a
poor diet will contribute. So a diet rich in nutrients and
relatively free from potential chemical hazards such as
pesticide and processing residues is likely to be beneficial.
But such a diet should be followed by everyone who values
their health, and there is no need to use a synthetic form.
Choosing nutritious natural foods instead of processed junk
food is the best solution.

Turning your body into a sort of unnatural chemical
factory can provoke a disaster when you have to go back to
proper food. It is far better to stay with natural food and
avoid the dangers.

Very-low-calorie Diets:
Summary

MODE OF ACTION

Starvation-level input leads to rapid glycogen and water loss followed by continuing loss of both fat and lean tissue.

CLAIMED BENEFITS

Rapid weight loss.

Full nutrient range allows long-term use.

Reduced hunger.

Convenient and easy to use.

Guidance from 'counsellor'.

DRAWBACKS

Product unpleasantness; may cause vomiting and other side-effects.

Some users experience ravenous hunger.

Metabolic depression.

Fatigue, fainting common.

Dieter loses social contact of shared meals.

Monotony.

Very rapid weight regain on return to normal food.

No learning of improved eating habits.

POTENTIAL DANGERS

Progressive, possibly irreversible loss of lean tissue with each return to diet means metabolic rate continues to fall while dieter grows flabbier.

Long-term risk of malnutrition due to missing trace nutrients.

Very rapid weight loss may cause serious illness.

CHAPTER 4

Low-carbohydrate Diets

Low carbohydrate diets are the favourites for promotion by members of the medical profession. Almost every weight-loss system with pretensions to medical acceptability has been a low-carbohydrate method. The most famous is *The Scarsdale Medical Diet*, developed by Herman Tarnower, MD; related diets have been produced by Drs Stillman (*The Doctor's Quick Weight Loss Diet*), Atkins (*Calories Don't Count*), Mackarness, Pennington and other medical practitioners. Occasionally a version of this type of diet appears without recourse to medical pretensions; Margaret Danbrot's *4-Day Wonder Diet* is an example.

The medical preoccupation with low-carbohydrate dieting is a curious phenomenon in view of the many hazards of this approach to weight loss. This method disrupts the metabolic processes of the body in ways that are bound to impair health.

What all these diets share is a very low proportion of carbohydrate. Carbohydrate is the major food component that we get from plants, which create it from carbon dioxide, water and energy from sunlight; it includes starches and sugars, and all our bulky foods such as grains, vegetables and fruit.

Low-carbohydrate slimming diets are also low in calories, though part of their sales patter may be the suggestion that they do not require calorie control. Forms vary in the different foods that are substituted for carbohydrates; earlier versions tended to be high-fat diets (*The Drinking Man's Diet* and others that were similar), while high-protein diets came to predominate as medical opinion turned against fat in recent years.

Cutting carbohydrate out of the diet induces metabolic changes that cause spectacular weight loss, mainly by causing a rapid loss of body water. These diets cause large amounts of hazardous wastes to be produced and water is drawn out of the body tissues to allow removal of these wastes. Much of the protein in a low-carbohydrate diet cannot be used by the body, so it is broken down into urea. Metabolising protein in this way makes some energy available to compensate for the lack of carbohydrate, which is the body's preferred energy source. But humans can only tolerate a small amount of urea; it must be quickly removed in the urine, so urine production is accelerated.

When healthy body tissues are broken down to make up for the inadequate intake of nutrients in these diets, the problem is compounded. The muscles need carbohydrate to burn fat, and when this is not available, the body will sacrifice lean tissue – even though there may be an excess of protein in the diet. This adds to the water loss and the general hazard of low-carbohydrate dieting.

Yet more water is lost when the body burns glycogen, its only readily available source of carbohydrate. This is stored in the liver and the muscles, in combination with water. So as glycogen is burnt and not replaced, more urine is produced.

The spectacular weight loss that occurs in the first week of a low-carbohydrate diet is therefore entirely predictable – but it represents a negligible loss of fat. As the dieter flushes body water and essential minerals down the lavatory, the scales show a steady loss of pounds. Unfortunately, scales are unable to distinguish between fat and water: a pound of one weighs precisely the same as a pound of the other.

Struggling to function in the absence of essential carbohydrates, the body will try to burn fat, but it requires carbohydrate to metabolise it completely. Within a few days on a low-carbohydrate diet, the products of incomplete fat metabolism, known as ketone bodies, begin to accumulate in the blood, causing a condition called ketosis. The most obvious early symptom is foul-smelling breath, often with a strong suggestion of nail varnish remover. Ketosis is said by some diet authors to increase the rate at which fat is burnt but, in fact, physiologists have proved in careful experiments that the reverse is true; ketosis slows down the rate of fat loss. When fat cannot be metabolised efficiently, the body tends to avoid using it; muscular activity is inhibited and the body's metabolic rate falls. Sustained activity is impossible when you are in ketosis.

Severe ketosis is very damaging. It can happen whenever there is too little carbohydrate in the diet, though its most savage form is peculiar to untreated diabetes, when lack of insulin makes carbohydrate unavailable to the cells. Rapid wasting occurs; dehydration is followed by loss of muscle tissue. Even a short episode of ketosis can produce lasting effects in diabetics, especially if it occurs at the same time as muscular effort, when the muscles involved will be damaged.

Diet authors seem to imagine that ketosis is only damaging for diabetics, although no rationale is offered for this assumption. Instead, dieters are encouraged to believe that ketosis is a desirable state because it is associated with reduced appetite and weight loss. Herman Tarnower, originator of the Scarsdale Diet, has this to say of ketones: 'If you are producing them, it is a sign that your body is burning off fat at an accelerated rate; you are enjoying *Fast Fat Metabolism*.' But as we have explained, this is totally wrong. The weight lost is not fat, but water and glycogen; then, if the diet continues, there is a potentially hazardous loss of lean tissue.

Some diet authors have suggested that the elimination of ketone bodies in the urine itself leads to a significant loss of calories. This has been measured; it accounts for 150 calories a day at most.

The greatest hazard of any low-carbohydrate diet is probably the increased risk of serious heart disease. We believe that this type of diet could even precipitate heart attacks – especially among the severely overweight men who seem to favour this high-meat style of eating. This danger is due to the interaction of a range of factors including disturbances of the blood chemistry and exhaustion; and obese people are particularly susceptible to heart problems.

Metabolic effects that put the heart at risk include the accumulation of uric acid in the blood and falls in potassium, magnesium and calcium levels caused by increased urine production. Together these changes increase the risk of potentially fatal heart rhythm disturbances. At the same time, the concentration of fat in the blood may be increased, adding another cardiac risk factor.

Extreme fatigue and fainting are common with low-carbohydrate diets. Characteristically, the authors of the diets minimise the significance of these problems. But the risk of a heart attack (as well as other illness) is greatly increased by exhaustion. Any diet that produces physical exhaustion is potentially hazardous, especially for over-weight people, who are prone to heart disease. Many are encouraged to lose weight in order to reduce their risk of heart problems; it is a tragic irony that a low-carbohydrate diet could just precipitate the feared heart attack.

Disturbed fat metabolism damages other body systems too. The gall bladder and the pancreas can be affected, and inflammation of either organ can occur during the diet or shortly afterwards. Pancreatitis can be fatal.

The increased flow of concentrated urine produces another set of hazards. Not only are essential minerals such as potassium lost, but the kidneys are put under strain as the load on them is increased. The kidneys themselves can suffer, and kidney stones may be formed. These produce one of the most excruciating pains known to humanity and can cause lasting damage to the kidneys and urinary system. When the kidneys are unable to remove the overload of urea sufficiently quickly, a high protein diet can precipitate gout. This painful condition is due to the formation of crystals of the urea in the joints; it occurs when the uric acid concentration in the blood is too high.

The low bulk, low-fibre content of these diets leads to yet another set of potential problems, this time with the intestine. Constipation is the first warning symptom. This is not taken seriously by Dr Tarnower, who writes, 'As one gets older, the need for a laxative is not unusual. I have patients who have taken a senna preparation every day for over 30 years, with very satisfactory results.' Most doctors would disagree strongly with this dismissive attitude; regular use of laxative preparations should be avoided because it can seriously damage the bowel. Diets that cause constipation are also associated with increased risk of many types of illness, ranging from cardiovascular disease to cancer of the colon. Hazards of long-term reliance on low-carbohydrate, low-fibre diets include a range of serious intestinal diseases, including diverticulitis (inflammation of the wall of the bowel) and appendicitis.

Fibre is but one of the essential dietary components that these diets lack. Essential fatty acids are mainly derived from the plant foods that are specifically excluded from low-carbohydrate diets, so they too may be missing. Low-fat forms of these diets usually forbid foods such as cooking oils, oil-based salad dressings, oily fish, nuts and avocado, all rich in the fats that are necessary for good health. Many people do not get enough of these crucial nutrients in normal circumstances; adopting a diet in which they are in even shorter supply could be enough to precipitate illness.

The consequence can be a multi-faceted illness which affects all body systems because essential fatty acids are involved in regulatory processes in many metabolic chains. Shortage of them can damage the skin, joints, nervous system and immune system, increasing the risk of common diseases of our culture such as allergies and arthritis. Early warning signs include rough and scaly skin, nervous problems and bowel disease.

The Scarsdale Medical Diet is so replete with references to its originator's medical qualifications and practice that most readers would probably be astonished that the diet could be so hazardous. Potential problems are theoretically reduced by the warning that the strict diet should not be followed for more than two weeks at a time. During the next two weeks, dieters are expected to follow 'keep-trim eating', which allows a somewhat wider variety of foods. But this is still a low-carbohydrate diet, and whilst its passable balance means that some of the most severe effects are avoided, it will not provide the energy necessary for more than minimal physical activity.

Adding carbohydrate to the diet will immediately cause weight to be regained. Water will be re-absorbed into the tissues, and the apparent advantages of the diet disappear. After a period on a high protein diet, normal eating always causes weight gain. It is just another form of the diet seesaw.

The sheer unpleasantness of a low-carbohydrate diet should be enough to dissuade anyone from adopting it; but when dieting is accepted by guilt-laden fat people as the punishment they feel they deserve for previous over-indulgence, a miserable regime will be tolerated. The comments of the American comedienne Renee Taylor on the Scarsdale diet seem particularly apt: 'I lost weight, but as soon as I went off the diet I gained again. Later on I felt sympathy for Jean Harris [Dr Tarnower's mistress: she shot him]. She should have put Dr Tarnower in a room and made him go on his own diet. That would have been punishment enough.' (Quoted from *My Life on a Diet*, G. P. Putnam's Sons, New York, 1986.)

There is no particular group of people for whom this type of diet is suitable, only groups for whom it is particularly dangerous. We believe that the Scarsdale diet and others like it should never be used, even for short periods. They have no advantages to balance their undoubted risks.

Low-carbohydrate Diets
(e.g. The Scarsdale Diet): Summary

MODE OF ACTION
Induce ketosis, glycogen and water loss.
Low energy input leads to loss of fat and lean tissue.

CLAIMED BENEFITS
Rapid weight loss.
Reduced hunger.

DRAWBACKS
Weight loss slows after first week; rapid regain when carbohydrate included in diet.
Unappetising regime.
Fatigue, lack of stamina.
Metabolic depression.
Halitosis.
Constipation.

POTENTIAL DANGERS
Nutritional imbalance; inadequate intake of essential nutrients could cause malnutrition.
Potentially fatal risk to heart, kidneys and other organs.
Excessive waste production may precipitate kidney stones, gout, pancreatitis.
Diet type linked with cancer.

CHAPTER 5

Tropical Fruit Diets

By far the most successful diet of this genre is *The Beverly Hills Diet*. Sold as the secret of the Hollywood stars, the diet was created by Judy Mazel, who has singlemindedly built a cult around the pineapple.

For Ms Mazel, dieting is a way of life, and her particular diet 'the key to happiness', 'a dream come true'. To us, her book reads like a primer in anorexia.

The Beverly Hills Diet is a curious and original mixture of wild assertions, patently inaccurate pseudo-science, gimmicks and quasi-religious exhortation. Heavily disguised behind all this is a system which relies on a very low calorie intake on most days. Calories are said to be irrelevant to the diet because it permits unlimited quantities of particular foods; you can (in theory) eat all day on the Beverly Hills Diet. However, since only one or two foods (usually pineapple or watermelon) may be permitted for the whole day, it is very difficult to achieve a high calorie intake. We estimate that a Beverly Hills dieter will consume an average of well under 1000 calories a day on this most unbalanced of diets.

The emphasis on tropical fruit characterises this diet from Day 1, when you are permitted only pineapple until evening, when you may indulge in two bananas. On Day 2, you get papaya with mango in the evening. On Day 3 it's papaya and pineapple, Day 4 watermelon only. The sequence continues with more fruit into the second week: grapes only on Days 9 and 10; but on Day 11 it changes. You are allowed 8 oz of bread and three ears of sweetcorn,

with butter! But do not get too excited about this indulgence; it's all you are allowed to eat that day and you will
be back on the pineapple on Day 12.

These drastic limitations continue for the six weeks of
the Diet. On Day 37, you get pineapple, followed by
strawberries in the evening – nothing else. Day 38: watermelon. Day 39: papaya ... but you can have a Chinese,
Japanese or Middle Eastern (not Mexican or Italian)
dinner! On Day 40 you pay for the dinner with a day on
watermelon only. And this is the way the system continues:
eat a meal one day, fast on a single fruit the next.

The rationale for Ms Mazel's obsession with fruit has
nothing to do with the combination of few calories with
relatively high bulk, palatability and convenience which
makes it the preferred type of food for many calorie-
conscious people. She focusses on the supposed value of
enzymes in the particular types of fruit chosen for each
day. Papaya and pineapple are said to contain particularly
efficient fat-burning enzymes. Watermelon is said to have
special cleansing properties. Each fruit is selected and the
sequence designed to produce a particular effect on the
body.

Ms Mazel's discussion of the qualities of these fruits in
relation to weight loss makes fascinating reading. We learn,
for example, that pineapples and strawberries contain an
enzyme (bromaline) which 'actuates the hydrochloric acid
in your stomach and helps to burn up the fat'. This is
nonsense. Hydrochloric acid in the stomach needs no
'actuating' and plays no part in burning body fat. Many
foods do indeed contain enzymes which have a range of
functions; enzymes in fruits can make them taste sweeter
than they otherwise would, which is why cooking fruit and
denaturing its enzymes often makes it taste sour. But they
do not have any fat-burning effect, and any link with
metabolising fat would certainly not be in the stomach.

Similar myths and misconceptions recur throughout the
book. We read, for example, that 'a single drop of syrup'

on a pancake 'neutralises the enzyme ptyalin', the component of saliva which breaks down starches. We wonder
where this idea originated; it certainly did not come from
scientific research. It makes no biochemical or biological
sense.

For all the pseudo-scientific explanation offered, Ms
Mazel gives no convincing justification for what she says,
apart from her own experience of weight loss and the
reports of successful slimming by various entertainers. But
no special enzyme effects would be required for weight loss
on a regime as restricted as the Beverly Hills Diet. The
system is bound to be effective as a method for weight loss
for those who can stick to it simply because it permits so
little food. For people who do as Ms Mazel does, effectively
starving themselves for two or three days a week in
perpetuity, the diet would probably continue to work. The
cost is chronic malnutrition and a deeply unhealthy obsession with food and weight.

Not that Ms Mazel sees her twin obsessions as unhealthy;
far from it. She does her best to encourage her readers to
become just as obsessive as herself. She urges readers to
'commit yourself to a daily love affair with your scale . . .
Make it your best friend and your lover . . . Love your scale
and embrace it; it is the key to your success and your
foundation to your sense of being.'

If Ms Mazel gains a pound on top of her usual 'ideal'
weight of 7 stone 4 pounds, she reverts to living on
pineapple, or watermelon, or whatever single fruit her
strange dietary system dictates. In her need for total control
over her intake and weight she behaves very much as an
anorexic does; if more happily and more successfully than
those who are unable to reach this point of satisfaction. The
health of her slimming business no doubt helps to keep her
from following the tragic road of the anorexic too far.

Ms Mazel fits neatly into the group of people, labelled
'secondary anorexics' by some psychologists, who use food
to satisfy emotional needs. She admits, 'I am still obsessive

and compulsive when it comes to food and eating. I still eat a triple order of potato pancakes without choking, an entire roast beef without blinking an eye, a whole, extra-rich cheesecake without a single gasp. I still respond to emotional situations by eating.' (p.144)

Rather than come to terms with herself by working through her problems with food and weight, Judy Mazel has successfully rationalised her obsessions. This is not unusual in anorexia, which is typically a problem of intelligent perfectionists. Many anorexics are deeply interested in nutrition, and will work out a whole system of justification for what is, in essence, a dangerous form of neurotic conversion.

Drawing on her lifetime study of eating problems, the psychotherapist Hilde Bruch describes anorexics who have systematically built up individual nutritional theories to support their relentless pursuit of thinness. One of her patients, having decided that chicken liver was the nearest to a perfect food, chose to live on two chicken livers a day. The fear of eating the tiniest morsel of foods seen as dangerous to the reducing diet is common among anorexics, who may wipe every mouthful of meat on absorbent paper to remove all traces of fat or gravy; there is a clear parallel with Ms Mazel's horror of a single drop of syrup on her pancake or a smidgen of protein with her potatoes.

The Nonphysical Exercises which form an important part of the regime reproduce typical anorexics' retorts to expressions of concern about what they do to themselves. Dieters are encouraged to dismiss any suggestion that they might be getting too thin. Anorexics characteristically feel better and more in control when they are starving themselves; the same is true of Judy Mazel. It is expressed clearly in the 'positive talkback' for Week Five, a list of proposed answers for concerned friends: 'Why should I stop doing something that makes me feel so good?'

Neurotic behaviour of any sort becomes self-perpetuating when it relieves anxiety. Self-starvation has the effect of relieving the fear of becoming fat which is Judy Mazel's preoccupation. However, it is undoubtedly dangerous – much more dangerous than over-eating. Admittedly, not many of those who are constantly dieting actually go so far as to starve themselves to death, but their health is certainly damaged. In her illuminating book, *Eating Disorders*, Hilde Bruch has much to say about the social pressures that create the twin extremes of extreme obesity and self-starvation. She is adamant that many can achieve slimness 'only at a great sacrifice of health and competence'. She compared death-rates of anorexics with those for the morbidly obese and found that extreme *fear* of fatness is much more hazardous than fatness itself.

Those whose fear of fatness took them into anorexia characteristically felt no concern about the damage that their refusal to eat was causing. The socially generated motivation to be thin was much stronger than internally generated hunger cues. Indeed, many anorexics deny that they feel hungry, although they are obsessed with food and recipes. Reading Judy Mazel's book alongside Dr Bruch's, the parallels between the two – one a report on anorexics and their attitudes, the other a diet book by a woman who, like others with the same problem, would surely deny her anorexia – are frighteningly obvious.

For Judy Mazel to hold pathologically distorted attitudes to her body is unfortunate; for her to endeavour to spread such attitudes among the public at large is tragic. Some of those who read *The Beverly Hills Diet* will be deeply susceptible to her message. Their lack of self-acceptance could be focussed and translated into full blown anorexia. Having a best-selling diet book as their guide to legitimise self-starvation, they will be set firmly on the road to illness and unhappiness.

Of course, most readers will not go along with Ms Mazel's way of thinking. For some individuals, experiencing the Beverly Hills Diet can actually have beneficial results – at least for a while. Peter, an overweight businessman who eats for the sensation of having something in his mouth, discovered that he feels better on fruit than rich foods and meat. Eating these things on different days in strict accordance with the directions in the book, he learnt how his body responded to different types of food. After six weeks on the diet, his eating habits were changed, and a year later he proudly told us that he had regained only about half the weight he had lost. However, Peter is a most unusual dieter whose use of food is more closely related to his constant desire to suck his thumb than to any nutritional needs.

For Peter, the value of the Beverly Hills Diet was in teaching him something about what food means to him and how it affects him. This is one of Ms Mazel's stated aims and it seems to be successful. What Ms Mazel does not allow is the next step: developing the ability to judge what and when to eat from internal cues. She insists that the scales, in combination with her esoteric rules, should fix what is eaten. It is not a healthy approach.

Using rules and fixed instructions in this way will appeal to some people with eating problems related to an inability to recognise internal cues to hunger or satiation. Many chronically overweight people will tend to eat all that is in front of them automatically, without questioning whether they actually want it; thinner people are usually more aware of their food needs and stop eating more readily when they are satisfied. Sometimes difficulty with internally generated cues leads to total reliance on social cues; Hilde Bruch reports on patients who would only eat when they could see another person (usually mother) eating, and then match that person, mouthful for mouthful. For such people, it may be a relief to abrogate responsibility for eating choices; following closely defined rules allows eating behaviour to be fixed by someone who is believed to have superior knowledge or understanding of what is required.

While difficulties with recognising and meeting their own food needs are common among people with weight problems related to inappropriate eating, giving them a fixed schedule of strictly limited types of food does little to help them overcome their problem. While some may discover, like Peter, that they can get as much emotional satisfaction from apples as from steak and kidney pudding, this knowledge may not be helpful for future maintenance of health and weight unless it is complemented by an understanding of the way needs for food change with time and circumstances. This sort of knowledge comes from exploration of one's own reactions to, and feelings about, food; from feeling free to select what one wants rather than adhering to any feeding schedule.

Of course, selection of food according to need and internally generated cues would defeat the object of the whole exercise for those who think in the same way as Judy Mazel. If your body functions best for the way you live when you weigh ten stone, but you are still trying to maintain yourself at a skinny eight stone, then you will have to overrule those internal cues. The problem here is one of attitude. If you are rejecting yourself and trying to remake yourself in a more supposedly desirable form, you may choose to ignore or override the internal cues that work to maintain you in your individual shape. By fixing your mind on the goal of inappropriate skinniness, it is possible to learn to ignore hunger pangs so completely that you cease to be consciously aware of them. This, we believe, is what Judy Mazel has done. It is a characteristic adaptation of anorexia.

The suppression of hunger that is essential to such a rigid regime as the Beverly Hills Diet need not be entirely psychological in origin. Among the many problems with this type of frankly cranky diet is that it is nutritionally imbalanced, and those who adhere to it are likely in course of time to suffer micronutrient deficiencies. Zinc deficiency is particularly probable because the fruit on which the diet relies is a poor source of zinc. This leads to loss of appetite and anorexia. So chronic undernutrition on a diet of this type can become self-perpetuating and turn into dangerous self-starvation.

The concept of a balanced diet is one which Ms Mazel finds worthless, and she has rejected it in favour of her own ideas about combining foods. She maintains that different foods cannot be digested properly unless some hours elapse between eating each one. Dieters are expected to eat nothing for a couple of hours between finishing the pineapple or other main food of the day, and starting on the bananas that they are permitted to eat before bed. On days when protein is permitted, no other type of food is allowed for the rest of the day. According to Ms Mazel, the body cannot digest anything else for many hours after protein has been eaten, and any other food will be transmuted directly into fat by some process that she does not explain. While the ideas described in *The Beverly Hills Diet* are more far-fetched than any other food-combining theories we have met, these others are based on similar principles. We discuss different diets based on food combining in Chapter 8, where we give our reasons for dismissing the theory.

While Ms Mazel ascribes particular fat-burning properties to tropical fruits such as pineapple and papaya, other diet-mongers have picked different fruits as the centrepieces of their diets. These are promoted as having special properties which supposedly make the diets work. We have been unable to find independent evidence for the value of any specific type of fruit in accelerating fat loss, although fruit does play a valuable role in a health-promoting diet.

Improved fat-burning is a property that has been attributed to grapefruit in particular, and various diets centred on the grapefruit have been developed. Like the Beverly Hills Diet, these in fact rely on severe calorie restriction for their effects, not some magic inherent in the grapefruit. Nevertheless, grapefruit (like papaya and other fruits venerated by Judy Mazel) is a rich source of nutrients and it has the special advantage of relative sourness. Eaten without sugar or other sweetener, grapefruit provides important nutrients, especially vitamin C and bioflavinoids (found in the pith of citrus fruits) without the rise in blood insulin levels that sweeter foods induce. People who eat fresh grapefruit in this way report that it helps reduce the desire for sweet food and thus regulates appetite in an enjoyable way. We find it delicious in its natural state and wonder why anyone should want to add to its sweetness.

Grapefruit juice does not confer the same benefits as fresh grapefruit. The flesh is also valuable and the whole fruit is far more satisfying than the juice alone.

The banana is another fruit that recurs in fruit-centred slimming diets. The rationale for reliance on bananas is less convincing. While they are high in some nutrients, notably potassium, they are not exceptionally so when compared with other types of fresh fruit and vegetables; and bananas can certainly induce an insulin rush that will hinder weight loss.

We believe that bananas are not notably useful in slimming diets. They became popular because they allow a return to babyhood: combined with milk, the sweet mush of a banana temporarily satisfies both emotional and physiological needs. Bananas are particularly attractive to the hungry because they provide instant gratification; however, hunger will return swiftly: the satiation provided by a banana does not last long.

So while you may enjoy bananas, do not imagine that they provide any special benefit. Eaten in quantity, they are more likely to lead to weight gain than loss. If you have adopted a high-energy lifestyle that includes bouts of intensive exercise, bananas can be very useful to top up energy stores; but if you fail to use the rapid-acting carbohydrate, they will contribute to your weight problem.

Apples are understandably popular as the basis for low-calorie diets because they provide bulk with few calories. Apple pectin has a particular value for urban people or those who live by busy roads, because it can clear the body of lead which is absorbed from car exhaust fumes. But living on apples may maintain your weight problem if you are particularly sensitive to the sprays used on them, or if you over-react to their sweetness and do not take sufficient exercise. Chapter 11 explains how pesticide residues can cause some people to gain weight.

It is particularly disturbing that fruit which is normally eaten whole and uncooked should be sprayed with poisonous chemicals up to two dozen times and, as if that were not enough, dipped in foul-tasting wax which cannot be removed by washing. Unsprayed apples may house the occasional maggot (though they need not, if proper biological methods of pest control are used) but they taste much better and have no destructive effects on our bodies.

Many diets that have fruit as a central feature refer to its cleansing effects on the body. Certainly the fresh clean taste of fruit gives the impression that it has cleansing properties, but there is more to it than this.

Dieters in mild ketosis will observe that one or two pieces of fruit can remove the foulness of their breath, de-coat their tongues and make their mouths taste much better. As a readily accessible form of carbohydrate, fruit can rebalance the system quickly, allowing complete metabolism of fat and other foods. It has been said that carbohydrate is the only truly clean-burning food because the only waste products are carbon dioxide and water. Without it, as we explained in the previous chapter, your body can become poisoned with its own waste products. So in this sense fruit does have a cleansing effect.

The nutrients found in fruit play other important detoxifying roles within the body. Vitamins A, C and E are crucial to effective de-toxification and some types of fruit are rich in all three. Wild fruit, eaten straight from the bush, is best of all: the vitamin content of wild blackberries, for example, can be six times that of cultivated blackberries.

Ripe fruit with deep-coloured flesh is particularly nutritious – and delicious.

Finally, fruit does have a cleansing effect on the intestine. Most types of fruit are rich in fibre and aid digestion. Fruit seems to be particularly important for protection from serious bowel diseases such as diverticulosis, which develop when the everyday diet contains insufficient bulk to move the bowel contents efficiently out of the body.

So some, at least, of the assertions made by those who propose fruit-based diets are justified. Fruit plays an important role in a health-promoting diet. But fruit will not maintain good health for long unless the diet is balanced with other types of food in sufficient quantity to meet all the needs of the body. It is not a good source of the nutrients we require for efficient carbohydrate metabolism, for example. It is a fallacy that fruit includes all that is necessary for its own metabolism in the body; in the long term, deficiencies will certainly develop. But in the short term, a day or so on fruit can be very beneficial, especially after a period of eating rich food.

Fruit is the one food that is specifically designed for eating. It grows to be eaten, and it develops sweetness so that we eat it when its seeds are ready to spread to other parts of the environment. Yet we should not be so completely seduced by the attractiveness of fruit that we attribute quasi-miraculous properties to it; remember, the fruit tree bears fruit for its own benefit – not for ours! It is not such a perfect food that we can use it as the central feature of our diet. Any diet that puts fruit in this position is likely to be bad for your health if you rely on it for more than a few days.

Tropical Fruit Diets: Summary

MODE OF ACTION
Severely limited food intake.
Dietary imbalance.

CLAIMED BENEFITS
Enzyme action of fruits said to facilitate fat loss.

Teaches user about effects of individual foods on the body.

A way of living for lifetime slimmers.

DRAWBACKS
Inadequate provision for nutritional needs.

Trace elements lacking, especially zinc.

POTENTIAL DANGERS
Malnutrition.

Gum disease, loss of teeth.

Anorexia.

CHAPTER 6

High-fibre Dieting

Audrey Eyton's *The F-Plan* is Britain's most successful slimming book. More copies have been sold than of any other diet book published in the country. High-fibre dieting quickly became popular and it won the support of many members of the medical profession. This was because it incorporated an idea which had considerable backing from nutritionists and doctors, without questioning the accepted slimming wisdom of calorie control.

The book emphasised the fact that our bodies cannot function well without much larger quantities of fibre than the average processed and de-natured Western diet contains. All plant foods contain fibre, which is a crucial component of plants; but milling removes it from refined products such as white flour. Audrey Eyton went further than the doctors in her discussion of the special properties of dietary fibre, but her book built on established medical assumptions and proposed a way of eating that was neither cranky nor wildly unbalanced.

While the supposed weight-removing properties of dietary fibre are emphasised in *The F-Plan*, the method does not pretend to rely solely on this. Ms Eyton maintains that, with her style of dieting, food calories are excreted unused. However, this dubious assertion is of minor significance because the F-Plan Diet is acknowledged to be a system of calorie-controlled eating in which weight loss is the consequence of reduced food intake.

Calorie counting alone, however, is not enough for a best-selling diet book. There has to be the gimmick, the amazing extra ingredient or special feature peculiar to the system that can be said to cause the body to shed fat faster and less painfully. A recurring characteristic of diet systems is the over-selling of the gimmick, and the oversell of fibre in Ms Eyton's book fits neatly into the familiar pattern.

Two crucial half-truths recur in *The F-Plan*. The first is that you can avoid feeling hungry if you fill your belly with high-fibre foods such as bran. The second is that doing so will prevent absorption of some of the calories in the food you eat. Both rely on a simplistic view of ourselves that does not fit reality.

The role of an empty belly in producing the sensation of hunger is one that has been investigated by psychologists and physiologists for almost a century. The results of their experiments show that having a substantial bulk filling one's stomach or intestine is not sufficient to prevent the sensation of hunger. If the bulk provides no nutrition – for example, diet aids based on such substances as methyl-cellulose – it usually makes no difference whatever to the perception of hunger. The brain is not easily fooled by manoeuvres of this kind; even if filling yourself with bulk seems to work once or twice, any suppression of appetite will be merely temporary and the effect will quickly be lost.

For overweight people, whether the stomach feels full or empty has especially little relevance. This was demonstrated in a series of neat experiments by the psychologist Stanley Schachter of Columbia University. In one experiment, he persuaded a group of volunteers to swallow a small balloon designed to record hunger contractions in their stomachs. He found that whereas 70 per cent of slim people felt hungry when their stomachs contracted, less than half of the overweight volunteers associated hunger with contractions. For them, the sight of food or the passage of time since the last meal was more likely to stimulate eating. And while a full stomach would be a potent signal for slim people to stop eating, it did not have the same effect on the fat group. They tended to eat so fast that the brain would not signal that they had had enough until they had consumed more than they needed.

Bran is the main source of bulky fibre recommended in *The F-Plan*. Dieters are persuaded that a mixture of bran flakes, bran buds and bran, with a sprinkling of dried fruit and chopped almonds, will be sufficient to keep them satisfied for many hours. Every day, the diet is supplemented by just under three ounces of this mixture, to be eaten with skimmed milk to ward off hunger.

The problem is that, in reality, the exceptional virtues of 'fibre-filler' do not meet the expectations that Ms Eyton builds up. Chronically undernourished dieters will continue to feel hungry even after a serving of this mixture. Even those who are not undernourished but lead an active life will find it inadequate. This is because hunger tends to continue while the body's nutritional needs remain unmet – and a portion of fibre-filler will not be enough to meet anyone's needs for long.

It may seem to satisfy at first. In addition to bran, fibre-filler contains sugar in dried fruit and in sweetened cereals such as All-Bran which will take the edge off hunger, especially in combination with milk. Some effects may last a little longer; high-fibre diets reduce fluctuations of blood sugar which are associated with both hunger and fat deposition. But soluble fibre such as that found in oatmeal is actually more effective than wheat bran, so Ms Eyton's mixture is not ideal even for the purpose for which she designed it. Unsweetened muesli generally has greater nutritional value and contains fibre of a more useful type.

The idea that fibre prevents absorption of some of the calories in food may be a good sales gimmick but its relevance to weight loss is negligible. To the naive dieter it may appear to be confirmed by the increase in volume of the stools that happens as a natural consequence of remedying the severe deficiency in fibre that is common to people who live on a processed diet, low in bulky carbohydrate; but this increased volume is mainly water, along with some plant components that the human gut cannot break down and use.

Fibre comes in many forms. Most of us visualise woody substances like wheat bran or cabbage stalks, but in fact the term includes gums and pectin, materials which are not at all fibrous in the normal sense of the word. When scientists first began to recognise the importance of fibre in our diet, they tended to assume that there was only one type, and that all fibre just passed through the body unchanged, providing bulk to improve bowel action and nothing else. Not long ago, people used to talk about 'roughage', which one imagined had a sort of scouring action.

Today many nutritionists define fibre as the food components which pass through the stomach and small intestine undigested. In the large intestine, they are processed – by bacteria which live in our bodies in symbiotic harmony, breaking down substances with which we would otherwise be unable to cope and providing us (and themselves) with nutrients derived from them. These beneficial bacteria are now known to be very important in protecting us from bowel disease; when we fail to feed them properly with the carbohydrates they require, they may be largely replaced by potentially dangerous organisms. Bowel cancers and diseases ranging from appendicitis to diverticulitis are associated with this sort of change in the intestinal population. Instead of improving our nutritional status, as the symbiotic bacteria do, these unfriendly organisms can change fats and other food residues into bowel carcinogens.

So fibre does far more than simply carry the remains of our food through the gut. Far from depriving us of food, it actually helps to feed us even though we cannot digest it without bacterial help.

While natural plant fibre, eaten with the rest of the food in which it occurs, is essential to our good health, there has been some concern about the sort of *processed* fibre advocated in *The F-Plan*. Wheat bran contains. phytin, which some scientists believe interferes with absorption of essential minerals from our food. This is a controversial issue, yet to be resolved. It may be that the body adapts to a high intake of phytin, but it does seem that mineral availability falls at first with a high-phytin diet. This is likely to be particularly hazardous for habitual dieters, whose mineral status is usually poor because of chronically inadequate nutrition.

Some of the menus suggested by Ms Eyton for F-Plan dieters will actually compound the problem of mineral loss, for the diet includes many processed foods which are notoriously poor sources of trace nutrients. People subsisting on low-calorie diets need to choose foods which have a high nutritional value in relation to their calorie content; even without questioning the theoretical basis of this type of diet, it makes little sense to throw scarce food calories away on sausages and sugar. Yet many of the foods suggested contain added sugar; there is a whole section in the book devoted to stewed fruit desserts, each with its added helping of empty calories in the form of granulated sugar; and Ms Eyton's much-lauded baked beans are usually loaded with it.

This diet is designed to appear radical without actually proposing real changes in the eating patterns which contribute to weight gain. For those whose everyday diet is very poor, it offers some improvement; for example wholemeal bread, emphasised because of its fibre component, is nutritionally far superior to white; and the stuffed potato recipes are generally wholesome.

Like other low-calorie diets, the F-Plan is low in fat, which also represents an improvement over the standard British diet. But it is indeed unfortunate that Ms Eyton did not endeavour to convert her millions of readers to a simple wholefood diet which incorporates plenty of fibre without any special additions like 'fibre-fill', and which is free of empty calories.

A wholefood diet, rich in vegetables and whole grains, is naturally high in fibre and also rich in trace nutrients. Junk food like instant mash, pork sausage, sweet pickle, crisps and sugar does not contribute to good health. Yet these are part of the F-Plan diet!

The major problem of the F-Plan is under-nutrition. For those who try to live on it, the subjective effect will be hunger. This problem is minimised in the book – as it is in every diet book. The nearest we could find to a reference to the hunger that dieters experience was this comment: 'All slimming diets – the F-Plan included – require some degree of conscious effort and self-control . . . The essential reward for the dieter is that weekly weight loss.'

Unfortunately, the F-Plan produces the same sort of metabolic depression as any other low-calorie diet. That weekly weight loss will decline while the hunger remains. Dieters have told us that the method seemed to work beautifully the first time they tried it – but the second or third time, it was disappointing. Even the promise of a weekly weight loss can be broken for chronic dieters, whose bodies adapt as readily to the F-Plan as to any other form of calorie deprivation.

Perhaps more worrying are the effects on dieters whose already low zinc stores are depleted further through the action of phytin. For them, the problem may not be hunger but loss of appetite – anorexia related to zinc deficiency. Using massive quantities of fibre to achieve laxative effects, they could put themselves in a position analogous to those who abuse laxatives. Under these circumstances, mineral depletion can be increased as minerals are lost from the intestine. Accelerated removal of food from the body is a familiar strategy for many anorexics; and while the F-Plan does not point as clearly down that dangerous road as the Beverly Hills Diet, it could contribute to the problem of anorexia.

So while Audrey Eyton is absolutely right to promote the benefits of fibre in the diet, we do wish that she had put her proposals into a more healthy context! Eating plenty of fibre-rich complex carbohydrate is part of the healthy way to a slim body . . . but it makes no sense to us to add processed fibre to an already over-processed diet. We should be correcting our dietary imbalances by changing the basics, not by fiddling about with superficial adjustments and panaceas.

High-fibre Diets (The F-Plan): Summary

MODE OF ACTION
Low energy input.

CLAIMED BENEFITS
Healthy way of slimming.
Fibre said to satisfy hunger.

DRAWBACKS
Insufficient trace nutrients.
May reduce mineral absorption.
Diet loses effectiveness over time.

POTENTIAL DANGERS
Perpetual slimming alternating with regain.

CHAPTER 7

Calorie-counting Diets

Almost every person with a weight problem has tried counting calories. The second generation of calorie counters are already teaching their daughters their beliefs about foods they imagine are fattening or not; which are 'naughty' and which boringly commendable. Although calorie awareness peaks among figure-conscious women in their early twenties, almost half the population regularly use reduced-calorie foods marketed for slimmers. The 'one calorie' sales line of the diet soft drink ad has enormous appeal.

There are as many varieties of low-calorie diet as there are individuals counting calories; but the principle is always the same. An effective slimming diet, the authorities agree, is one which delivers fewer calories than the dieter uses up. Most people are convinced that calorie restriction is the only way to shed excess weight.

Calorie control is fundamental to all the diets we have studied. Although many of the bestsellers fail to acknowledge that calorie restriction is their crucial feature, other authors and organisations are more candid about what they offer. They operate on the belief that we grow fat because we regularly consume too many calories, and the only way to shed that fat is through a drastic cutback. This, they will admit, is an unpleasant process which requires considerable willpower; but they urge fatties to persevere or endure a lifetime of ugly and unhealthy flabbiness.

Implicit in all this is the assumption that people get fat because they are weak-willed, greedy and self-indulgent; so calls for greater self-control are readily accepted as appropriate. Overweight people pick up the covert message, adding an increment of guilt and self-disgust to their already poor self-image.

When a straightforward mismatch between calorie input and calorie expenditure is pinpointed as the source of the problem, there would seem to be two possible strategies for correcting the balance. One would be to cut input, the other to increase output. But dietmongers are pessimistic about the value of increasing output, largely on the grounds that burning calories through activity is said to be slow and inefficient.

Numerous popular authors quote figures for calorie use by activity that are designed to persuade readers that it is almost impossible to lose weight by adjusting the output side of the equation. For example, we learn from Dr Herman Tarnower (*The Scarsdale Medical Diet*) that 'A half-hour of energetic bicycling . . . uses up 200–280 calories, which you put right back on by eating an iced cupcake.' (p.164) Even a half-hour stint of stair-climbing – a feat of physical endurance, as anyone who has tried climbing long flights of stairs will know – is said to use up a maximum of 160 calories. That's a lot of pain for very little gain. For those who believe this, a reduced calorie diet seems much easier.

For decades, well-meaning people and less scrupulous individuals with an eye for a ready market have been designing different diets which are intended to make calorie control less miserable for slimmers. These appear at frequent intervals in magazines and books; they form the backbone of the regimes touted at slimming clubs; they are offered in the form of diet sheets by hospitals and doctors, clinics and nutritionists.

The other side of the coin for all these authorities is the view of the fat person as someone who regularly and needlessly overeats. After all, if you are taking in more calories than you need, it stands to reason – surely – that you must be overeating. The slimmer may protest that she eats much less than anyone else in the family, and the weight persists despite this; but many doctors and nutritionists will simply refuse to believe her, preferring to assume that she lies or is incapable of working out her actual calorie intake.

Many slimmers internalise assumptions of this sort. Eating makes them feel guilty: being so fat, they should not be eating. Yet their fat does not stop them from feeling hungry. Meals are made miserable by emotional conflict, celebrations spoilt by the ever-present awareness of the mounting calories and the inevitable deposition of flabby pounds on tummy, hips and thighs. For all that the diet authors say you can go to a restaurant and order your grilled fish without butter or sauce and your fruit salad without cream, you know that the whole point of enjoying the chef's food will be lost when you cannot eat it in its intended form. Others enjoy; the dieter exercises self-control – and suffers.

It's unfair, it's depressing, and it's no fun for the rest of the company either when you won't join in with the eating because you're locked into the misery of counting calories.

Counting calories becomes an obsession. Before long, most dieters know the calorie content of just about everything they eat. Calorie calculations fill the margins of students' lecture notes, cover old envelopes, notebooks and diaries. Portions are judged and weighed with the greatest care lest the total permitted for the day be exceeded. Food-substitutes like synthetic sweeteners and watered-down apologies for butter are avidly bought because they fit within the rules, even if they disappoint the palate.

Since, according to those who believe in the calorie-counting formula, one calorie is precisely the same as another, a calorie counter can select any pattern of diet as long as the total remains below the chosen figure. Predictably, young women, who are most obsessed with their diet and least concerned for their health, miss nutritious meals because they are dieting, and fill up with chocolate bars and over-processed snacks when hunger overcomes them.

Excessive coffee and cigarettes support the effort, adding to the health damage. This is the characteristic style of dieting among students and young people.

Calorie counting encourages people to put off eating until later because it is easier to resist food when you are not yet particularly hungry. But internal pressure to eat builds up to unbearable levels as blood sugar falls. This generates the style of chaotic dieting in which the day starts with black coffee for breakfast, more coffee for elevenses, biscuits and a small cube of low-fat cheese for lunch . . . and a mid-afternoon Mars Bar when self-control snaps. Then the calorie-count is re-instituted, restricting supper to permit an acceptable total for the day. By bed-time the belly is empty, the body restless. Sleep comes with difficulty to dieters.

Each day becomes a seesaw of starvation followed by desperation eating; the apparent logic of the system is destroyed by the stronger imperatives of the body. The mini daily seesaw becomes part of the larger seesaw of weight loss and regain that produces the seemingly inexorable increase in fatness that characterises long-term dieters.

For a short while, previously well-nourished young people will seem to do well enough on such a nutritionally deprived schedule as this. But as the battle against weight gain continues over years, the health costs begin to show. Pre-menstrual tension, poor skin, dark circles under the eyes, frequent infections – all these and more can be the consequences of micronutrient deficiency due to ill-judged calorie counting. Constant attention to an aspect of food that is effectively irrelevant to the selection of a balanced diet means that important nutritional issues are ignored.

It is a distortion of eating behaviour that produces other behavioural distortions in its wake.

As time goes on, the situation gets worse in every way. Even if the dieter tries to go about calorie restriction in a sensible way, cutting out foods which offer poor nutritional value in relation to their calorie content, the law of diminishing returns in slimming diets will operate against her. And the longer the dieting continues, the more dramatic are the effects of a fall from grace. Breaking the diet, going for those biscuits and chocolate and cakes, will be disastrous. The pounds will come roaring back.

Despair brings on the binge. The poor dieter stuffs herself, no longer enjoying the forbidden foods that she missed so desperately, because the guilt that surrounds them (another 450 calories, my God, *why* am I doing this?) destroys their flavour. Yet somehow she is unable to stop.

And so she learns to make herself vomit.

This is the way that thousands of unfortunate women (and increasing numbers of young men) avoid the consequences of the almost inevitable binge that follows the self-deprivation of calorie restriction. It is a pattern that can quickly get completely out of control, causing progressive damage to the body. Bulimia – obsessive self-induced vomiting – is a dangerous and increasingly common form of anorexia.

For those who do not, or cannot, follow the dangerous road to bulimia, the long-term consequences of calorie restriction are still miserable. Weight loss gradually slows or even stops as metabolic depression sets in, with its effects of tiredness, weakness, vulnerability to cold and loss of enjoyment of more and more of the pleasures of life as the denial of appetite spreads its chilly influence.

Some people survive for years, sustained by fear of fatness. The champion jockey Lester Piggott kept himself perpetually half-starved and his body adjusted to it. But the rewards for his lightness were great. For most people, there are few rewards, just the constant rejection of self and the suppression of desire. Even the weight may stay stubbornly in place, for the calorie theory addresses only one of the functions of fat and that in a one-sided way. Calorie restriction is a totally negative process, based on denial, contributing nothing.

To sustain such a regime is extremely difficult; most long-term dieters feel they are fighting a losing battle. So support systems now exist to shore up flagging willpower.

The most popular form of support is the slimming group. Weight Watchers is the best known and most successful of these, though there are others, including those formed by slimming magazine publishers. While there are variations between different groups, and some differences between organisations, the principles on which they work are the same.

Slimming groups use social support to keep their members on the narrow path of calorie restriction. Slimmers are weighed at weekly meetings where their progress towards a goal weight is recorded. Those who lose weight will be warmly congratulated and bask in the admiration of other class members; while those who fail to lose will be questioned to find the reason for their problem and may be fined. Coffee, advice, information, discussion, and a short talk from the class leader, complete the picture.

Weight Watchers classes are led by ex-members who have lost weight with Weight Watchers and continue to maintain their goal weight. They are trained to take classes and given a topic for discussion each week. Inevitably, every group leader is different and her individual style will colour the class; but the general principles of weekly weighing and encouragement are to be found in every group.

Those who reach their goal weight can continue to go to Weight Watchers meetings without any charge for as long as they maintain their chosen weight. The organisation provides information to guide them in the perpetual food restriction that they rely on to stay slim.

The Weight Watchers system provides precise instructions on what dieters may eat each day. For example, breakfast in the first week is likely to be grapefruit or orange juice, 1 oz (28g) – weighed, please, ladies! – of cereal with skimmed milk or an egg and a slice of bread, plus tea or coffee. Lunch might be 3 oz (80g) canned fish with vegetables and/or salad and a thin slice of bread. Dinner will be 3 or 4 oz (80 or 110g) fish or meat with vegetables and a piece of fruit. A further piece of fruit and a natural yoghurt are usually permitted at any time during the day. Foods have to be weighed so that the quantities are precisely as permitted; the only exceptions are fresh, low-calorie vegetables such as green beans, broccoli, lettuce and celery, which are allowed in unlimited amounts. Dieters are advised to eat at least 6 oz (170g) of these vegetables each day.

This is a regime that provides about 1200 calories and a fairly high proportion of protein. Foods high in carbohydrate are drastically restricted; the slice of bread must weigh no more than one ounce (28g) and potatoes are not permitted, at least at first. Members are told to stick to the menu plan precisely and never to miss meals.

For some members, the method works admirably. A survey by the consumer magazine *Which?* found that more dieters had lost significant amounts of weight with the help of slimming clubs than in any other way. Encouragement for weight loss helps to maintain resolve in the face of the demands of appetite. The menu plan keeps the diet in passable balance, while the mild encouragement to increase activity levels might get some people moving when they would otherwise not have bothered.

For those few who change their lifestyles permanently in order to maintain their new slim figures, the results can last. One woman told me, 'It isn't a diet at all – you get as much food as you like.' Studying the menus, we could not agree – for those of us who like to eat half a large loaf every day, living on the Weight Watchers diet would be distinctly painful! Of course, many of those who lose weight regain it quickly when they return to their normal eating style – as they do when they give up any low-calorie regime. Some return repeatedly to Weight Watchers to shed the weight that they gain when they leave the group. As a long-term approach to slimming, it is very profitable for the organisation but not very effective for most of its members. Many pass through the groups but few continue coming, holding their goal weight to take advantage of the encouragement provided by the free classes.

Some people simply do not fit in with the assumptions of the group. They may find the ritual of regular public weighing and confession of dietary sins irksome. They may be unable to stick to a diet that does not permit satisfying snacks when they feel hungry. They may resent paying for knowledge that they feel they already have. They may rebel against the authoritarian structure. Or they may simply find that constant calorie restriction means that their target weight remains for ever out of reach because their metabolic rate is so depressed by perpetual dieting that their bodies will not shed that unwanted fat even when they adhere conscientiously to the rules. For them, the basic assumption of the slimming club – that the route to weight loss is the low-calorie diet – just does not work any longer. The social pressure merely adds to the load of misery that they already carry.

The underlying assumptions of the slimming clubs – that all weight above your 'target' is fat, that weight loss is all that is desired, and that calorie restriction is the only way to achieve it – are the fundamental problems with their approach. The social support can be valuable to members; what a pity it is so misdirected. What a pity it is used to refine and strengthen our society's already excessive pressure for unhealthy dieting. What a pity it reinforces the false idea that there is no alternative to calorie restriction. What a pity, in all, that misunderstanding of the nature of the slimming problem means that the potential value of the group is so often wasted.

We should not leave the topic of calorie-counting diets without considering the latest best-selling variant: Martin Katahn's *The Rotation Diet*. This system is said to overcome the metabolic depression caused by calorie restriction through a pattern of short-term drastic dieting followed by more lenient eating. The diet lasts for three weeks only, after which normal eating should be gradually resumed; then, after a break of at least a week, dieting can start again for another three weeks.

This is a particularly interesting book because its author, although advocating calorie restriction and selling the system as a diet, admits that the essential requirement for long-term success is *exercise*. 'Face the facts,' writes Dr Katahn on p.108. 'If you are sedentary, it will be almost impossible for you to manage your weight without finding some way to increase your activity level to the point that nature intended . . . Our bodies were designed for a high level of physical activity, and our appetites are matched to that level of activity.' On p.124 he makes the same point again. 'I cannot emphasise this too strongly: if you do not get active and stay active, you've got a snowball's chance in hell of maintaining any weight loss. You will face semi-starvation for the rest of your life if you remain sedentary and want to control your weight.'

We cannot quarrel with this! But we disagree that increasing metabolic rate through increased activity can reasonably be called 'dieting'. However, Dr Katahn, a psychologist, knows precisely what he's doing; his earlier book, *The 200 Calorie Solution*, advocated increased activity, not dieting, as the way to solve weight problems permanently. It was far less successful than *The Rotation Diet*. Dr Katahn has learnt from his experience of a market hooked on the illusion of low-calorie diets and quick weight loss regimes.

The low-calorie Rotation Diet itself is clearly designed to act as a psychological boost to slimmers by inducing quick weight losses at intervals during the long process of fat reduction through exercise. Its first effect will be water loss, achieved through severe sodium (salt) restriction combined with a strict 600-calorie high-protein diet with black coffee to increase diuresis. This part of the rotation is reminiscent of the Scarsdale Medical Diet (Chapter 4). After three days, 900 calories are permitted for the next four days, then 1200 calories a day for a week. The third week of the diet is like the first, with 600 calories followed by 900. These figures are for women; men get a more generous allowance of 1200/1500 calories for the first week, 1800 for the second, and 1200/1500 for the third and final week.

Regrettably, Dr Katahn does not appear to be as well informed about the physiological effects of this diet as about the necessity for exercise. He states on p.102 that the increased protein component of the diet will prevent loss of protein from the body. This is a fallacy that has been repeatedly disproved by scientific research. In his book on *Human Body Composition*, physiologist Gilbert Forbes discusses this research at some length. He states on page 70 that, 'It was shown many years ago that nitrogen (i.e. protein) balance cannot be maintained in the face of a subnormal energy intake regardless of the amount of protein fed.' He admits of only one exception to this rule, the hibernating bear. Humans, rats, birds, and all other creatures studied *always* lose protein when calorie intake is restricted, however much exercise they take.

Dr Katahn's assertion that the dietary component of this system does not reduce metabolic rate is impossible to test when it is not to be used without exercise. In his introduction to the diet on p.37 he hedges his argument with the warning that dieters must *'follow my instructions for maintenance'* (i.e. exercise every day); later on the same page, he repeats the exhortation: 'You must implement the entire plan.' We believe that sensitive people, especially regular dieters, *would* experience a reduction in metabolic rate if they followed the diet without implementing the exercise regime; but the system is too new for independent evidence to be available.

So is Dr Katahn's rotation diet really revolutionary? We do not believe so. As a long-term system, his dietary recommendations and comments on exercise are generally commendable; but the actual *diet* is just another variation on a familiar short-term weight-loss theme.

Calorie Counting: Summary

MODE OF ACTION
Low energy input.

CLAIMED BENEFITS
Can continue indefinitely.

DRAWBACKS
Obsession with calorie content of food.

Demands increasing willpower for diminishing rewards.

Falling metabolic rate.

May be inadequate carbohydrate for fat-burning activity.

Stop-start dieting produces increasingly flabby body.

POTENTIAL DANGERS
Malnutrition.

CHAPTER 8

Food-combining Diets

The theory of food combining, developed more than fifty years ago, is regularly revived by the designers of slimming diets. Some, like Judy Mazel, produce scarcely recognisable versions, but the recent American bestseller, *Fit for Life*, written by Harvey and Marilyn Diamond, and Leslie Kenton's *The Biogenic Diet* adhere quite closely to the classic form of the theory.

Basically, food combiners believe that different types of food cannot be digested at the same time, and by eating combinations like starch and protein – for example fish and chips, meat and potato, quiche, or cheese sandwiches – we prevent complete and efficient digestion. Weight gain is held to be one of the consequences of miscombining food, and weight loss results from conscientious adherence to food-combining rules.

Food-combining ideas originally evolved in a general health context. Dr William Hay, a general practitioner, developed the system in the early years of this century as a method of treatment for disease ranging from diabetes to arthritis. In Dr Hay's view, all disease was due to acid conditions in the body caused by inappropriate eating patterns, and his dietary rules were designed to restore the body's alkalinity.

The Hay System is described in detail in *Food Combining for Health* by Doris Grant and Jean Joice. It has five basic rules:

1. Starches and sugars should not be eaten with proteins and acid fruits at the same meal.

2. Vegetables, salads and fruit should form the major part of the diet.
3. Proteins, starches and fats should be eaten in small quantities.
4. Refined processed foods should be avoided.
5. At least four hours should elapse between meals of different character.

Although obesity is one of the many conditions said to be cured by the Hay system, weight loss is seen as an indirect consequence of improved health. Those who live by these dietary rules will, enthusiasts claim, move towards their ideal weight; excessively thin people will gain while fat people will lose. But neither Dr Hay nor the authors of *Food Combining for Health* emphasise this aspect of the diet. They comment that 'compatible eating is not recommended for people who are quite content with their state of health, or who can eat incompatible mixtures without discomfort or apparent harm.' (p.34) They do not claim that eating starch and protein in the same meal, for example, will upset everyone.

Those who suffer from frequent indigestion or other symptoms of excessive sensitivity to food do seem to benefit from the sort of careful combining advocated by Dr Hay and his followers. While the rationale for the system is not generally accepted by scientists, nutritionists or the medical profession, the balance of the diet is health-promoting and its many enthusiasts are convinced that it can confer great benefits. However, it is a low-energy diet that demands considerable self-discipline; it is likely to prove inadequate for many active people and unacceptable to gourmets.

Neither the Diamonds nor Leslie Kenton acknowledge the limitations of the Hay system. They deny that their diets produce weight loss because they are low in calories, though in fact they are. It would be difficult to consume more than about 1500 calories daily on either diet. Each advocates a way of eating that is both low in energy content and carefully and consciously controlled: The restrictions imposed on eating prevent casual indulgence in food as surely as the most rigid low-calorie diet. These are diets for the committed few.

Both the Diamonds' and Leslie Kenton's systems have a very large range of oppressive 'thou shalt nots', artfully hidden behind dietary rules that appear far more generous than they are. For example, both emphasise 'high water content' foods: fresh fruit and raw vegetables. Those who try a diet in which 70 per cent of food must be eaten raw quickly find that it is difficult to chew their way through enough to avoid losing weight and suffering the hunger that low-calorie dieters experience. Raw food diets produce weight loss whether they incorporate any deliberate combining or not. This is regarded as a problem with the Bristol Diet, designed for cancer sufferers who often need to gain weight. On raw food they are more likely to lose it.

This is not to suggest that raw foods are not beneficial for health, although we are doubtful about some of the claims made for them. It is absolutely true that most foods have the highest nutrient content when they are fresh and raw. In this state, they offer greatest benefit to the body. Cooking changes the nature of foods and the importance of such changes is not fully understood. It may well be true that denaturing some complex proteins reduces their value to the body. However, it is also definitely true that cooking can make other nutrients accessible to the body, and remove some hazards.

Cooked carrots, for example, have more available vitamin A than raw carrots. Well cooked grain and leavened breads contain less phytin, reducing problems with mineral absorption. Cooked egg white is safer to eat because the protein in raw egg white combines with some B vitamins, making them unavailable; people who eat large quantities of raw eggs have developed symptoms of severe vitamin deficiency. Many varieties of beans must be well cooked to prevent the illness that results from their consumption in the raw or undercooked state; the same is true of some root vegetables such as cassava.

A dramatic description of the effects of eating Mackenzie beans fresh from the plant appears in Lucy Irvine's story of life on a tropical island in *Castaway*. These beans are edible cooked but poisonous raw.

'By the time I had got back to camp I was full. I must have eaten at least two dozen beans raw ... Without any warning at all my bowels and stomach were suddenly squeezed with a grinding nausea. I felt dreadfully giddy ...

'My body became one convulsive organ of evacuation. After the first double-ended eruption, which had flooded the sand fore and aft with flowing pools, I just had the strength to move sideways to a clear patch before the next storm swept my guts ...'

Living on predominantly raw, fresh food (apart from beans, of course!) may be possible in tropical countries where such food is available all the year round and people do not have to cope with the rigours of cold weather, but for those who live in chilly countries with harsh winters it makes much less sense. This is something that many Californian diet designers fail to acknowledge, perhaps because it is outside their experience. Dietary requirements are not identical for different people living different kinds of lives, under different environmental conditions.

In this context, the Diamonds' assertion in *Fit for Life* that their dietary rules are consistent with the normal practice of the longest-lived races of the world is particularly strange. These people certainly do not rely on raw food – indeed, they would be unable to survive if they did! The Hunzakuts of the Himalayas, for example, live in a high valley which is snowbound for many months of the year. They do not enjoy year-round warm sunshine, nor do they have the benefit of heated greenhouses where fresh salads can be grown in winter. During the winter, they are forced to rely on stored and dried foods. While some grains and seeds can be restored to a fresh growing state by sprouting, the opportunity even for this is limited when houses have no central heating or airing cupboard in which seeds can spout and grow. In a cool home, damp seeds do not germinate and produce luscious sprouts; they just grow mouldy.

It was largely through the discovery of fire and the art of cooking that humans were able to colonise the temperate zones of the world. The frugivores of the tropics, both our own ancestors and the great apes who are our closest relatives, could not survive through a Northern winter on their raw fruit and seed diet. Evolution has led to many adaptations, in dietary needs as in other aspects of physiology, to allow humans to spread northwards even during the last great Ice Age. We have inherited these adaptations and we should acknowledge their relevance to our needs.

If human health and survival were dependent on a diet of raw foods, our species would be found only near the Equator and we should be very different. Pale-skinned humans would not exist at all. So while the Diamonds use evolutionary evidence to support their argument, they place an unfortunate reliance on data from very early ancestors, ignoring the adaptations that now characterise our race.

Some of the other proposals made by the Diamonds make even less sense when considered in an evolutionary context. Neither our ancestors nor the long-lived peoples of the world could have used *distilled* water for drinking, for example. Yet according to these authors, natural water is bad for our health. While we agree that tap-water is polluted and unpleasant to the taste, we cannot believe that pure spring water is inferior to flat, de-mineralised, distilled water. This seems to be something that we are expected to take on trust, since no evidence is offered. Unfortunately, such assertions merely serve to undermine our trust in other aspects of the thesis, which is a pity when the lifestyle described is a relatively healthy one and certainly superior to that of most slimming regimes.

Adding to the burden of disbelief inspired by *Fit for Life* are the assertions about the fate of miscombined foods. We learn that starch eaten with protein will ferment in the stomach, while the protein food putrefies. In this state, according to the food combiners, these foods become indigestible: 'Eating two concentrated foods (i.e. starch and protein) simultaneously will cause the food to rot, and rotten food CANNOT BE ASSIMILATED!' Eating two types of protein food at the same meal, apparently, will cause *both* to putrefy: an assertion which makes no sense even in terms of the justification for the theory given in the Diamonds' book. The problem with digestion had been explained as the consequence of the fact that proteins require an acid environment for digestion, while starches are digested more efficiently in an alkaline environment; so we would deduce that two proteins could be digested comfortably together. Not so, according to this theory.

How the protein manages to putrefy, a process that normally results from bacterial action, we are not told; similarly, we are not told how fruit or starch can ferment, when this process depends on the action of yeasts which would have great difficulty in surviving, let alone thriving and acting on our food, in the acid environment of the stomach. This is just another fairy story.

Even fruit, highly praised as the most valuable component of the diet described by the Diamonds, must be eaten with great care. 'UNQUESTIONABLY THE MOST IMPORTANT ASPECT OF FIT FOR LIFE' is that fruit must be 'eaten on an *empty* stomach.' (p.65) A cynical reader immediately suspects that the *empty stomach* is more important than anything that may be eaten. It could be the crucial feature of this diet, which is little more than semi-starvation in an elaborate disguise.

When we read the words, 'This is something that is easily verifiable' in the discussion of the way foods spoil and 'turn to acid' when miscombined, we went to the kitchen to test the theory with a horrific miscombination: cheese and tomato sandwiches. With its mixture of concentrated protein, starch *and* fruit, this should quickly produce the effects predicted by the Diamonds. But did the sandwiches cause us to 'run for medication', as these authors predicted? Of course not! Our appetites were satisfied in a most enjoyable way. We found it was very easy to disprove the theory. We do it every day, just like billions of other people throughout the world.

The emphasis on rotting and putrefaction is a clever way of putting people off eating. From a scientific point of view, it is sheer nonsense. Normal, efficient digestion of food in the human gut is not, in fact, fundamentally different from the processes of digestion by fungi or bacteria. All life-forms secrete digestive enzymes which break down food tissues; we just call the process 'rotting' when it results from fungal action, and 'putrefaction' when the organisms doing the digesting are bacteria. We give the same process a different label according to the circumstances under which it occurs. So the idea of ill-combined meals rotting or fermenting in the stomach is clearly designed to motivate readers through creating disgust at their own bodily processes, a strategy which will tend to undermine health and happiness.

If the assertions of the food combiners were valid, meals that contain protein-starch mixtures would not have developed independently throughout the world to become the staple way of eating for every human culture. Food combining theorists must condemn equally the eating patterns of the East, where fish, meat or eggs (concentrated protein foods) are eaten with rice, millet, wheat-flour pancakes and other starch foods, as well as the West, where we have potatoes, bread, pasta or other grain-based foods with our proteins.

This general style of eating has been prevalent throughout the temperate world ever since humans settled to agriculture and began to cultivate starchy crops and herd animals. Yet we have not been suffering thousands of years of indigestion, overweight and allergies as a consequence!

These problems have become prevalent only recently. Our lifestyle has changed in many ways, and the types of illness pinpointed by the food combiners have indeed resulted; but these recent changes did not include a move to new and dangerous patterns of food combining that would make the theory fit the facts of the real world.

Leslie Kenton's book, in many ways a much more intelligent exposition of the subject than *Fit for Life*, does not attempt to justify the Biogenic Diet in quite the same way, though the same arguments against the basic theory of food combining must apply. Nevertheless, she too proposes a diet that we believe is too insubstantial for people whose lives impose any more than minimal physical demands. Ms Kenton, whose determination to keep herself thin almost matches Judy Mazel's, manages to subsist on very little food and to go running too; this seems not to be enough to keep her sufficiently lean, for she fasts regularly, eating nothing but apples for one day each week.

Although Leslie Kenton maintains that she is not hungry on the Biogenic Diet, she has not achieved freedom from the desire for more substantial food. She warns readers to avoid more satisfying foods, on the grounds that hunger can be 'triggered' by eating them. Low-water-content foods, she writes, 'tend to increase cravings for more food and therefore force the slimmer to exert the most phenomenal willpower to keep from eating too much.' The cravings, clearly, are already there: the way to deal with them is never to permit yourself to give in.

Repeatedly she emphasises the warning, 'Never overeat'. This warning occurs so often that it raises questions in our minds – especially when the only foods you are allowed to eat on this diet are those which would not lead to fat deposition even if you had great platefuls at a sitting. We believe it reveals a chronic unsatisfied desire to eat a great deal more, firmly suppressed by a formidable will. Her diet demands four- or five-hour gaps between each meal, and does not permit snacks; such a regime inevitably produces hunger, tiredness and weakness. The risk for the dieter who attempts to follow in Ms Kenton's footsteps is the pattern of cravings, bingeing and self-punishing guilt that many already know all too well.

The principles on which both the Diamonds and Kenton agree are these: first, 70 per cent of the diet should be raw fruit and vegetables. Second, nothing but fruit is permitted before noon. Third, proteins and starches (with the exception of fresh vegetables) must not be eaten at the same meal; up to eight hours must elapse between eating these types of food. Both systems condemn all types of food additives and processed foods, as well as tea, coffee, alcohol and all drugs.

Both systems also emphasise the importance of frequent exercise. In Kenton's version, this must be strenuous exercise lasting at least forty minutes, at least four times a week. The Diamonds suggest a minimum of thirty minutes aerobic activity every day. The effects of both regimes would be much the same.

This level of regular exercise is in itself health-promoting and anyone who keeps to such a regime will quickly become quite slim. The problem is that it would be difficult for most people to maintain such a high level of energy output when the energy input level is so low – as it will inevitably be if the rules on combining and timing of meals are strictly adhered to.

So is there any point in following the food combining rules? We believe there is not. For people who experience particular difficulty with digestion, combining may perhaps be helpful; but since careful studies of such people reveal emotional tension to be the most important cause of indigestion, attending to this will be much more effective than adopting severely restricting dietary rules. The regular and extended aerobic exercise recommended by these authors would reduce emotional tension and would probably be sufficient in itself to overcome digestive problems.

The problem with adhering to the rules laid out in both these books is that common to all low-calorie dieting: hunger. When so many foods are prohibited, it would seem to many dieters that there is no way they can satisfy their hunger without breaking out of the system, which is far too inflexible and unresponsive to individual needs and fluctuations. This creates the temptation to snack on concentrated short-term energy foods like chocolate. The binge then follows, drawing its momentum from the combination of deprivation and self-disgust.

It is regrettable that the basically sensible dietary and lifestyle advice in both these books is overlaid with so much mystique and unconvincing theory. While this might make the books into talking-points that work well for publicity and sales, it makes them into impracticable life-guides. Trying to live by the rules laid down by the food combiners could make the struggle for slimness almost as miserable as it is under the regimes described in preceding chapters. Desires must be overruled; simple pleasure in eating becomes elusive. Part of the pleasure of a special dinner lies in the range of foods eaten together; but celebratory eating would be impossible for conscientous food combiners. This is a system that removes much enjoyment from life quite unnecessarily.

Food Combining (Biogenics): Summary

MODE OF ACTION
Low energy input.
Reduced intake of potential toxins.

CLAIMED BENEFITS
Health enhancement, reduction of allergies and cure for digestive problems.
Reduced risk of cardiovascular and other disease.
Long-term potential.

DRAWBACKS

Disruption of social and cultural eating patterns.

Demanding regime, difficult to sustain.

Unlikely to support very active life.

POTENTIAL DANGERS

None if sufficient food is eaten.

CHAPTER 9

Insight

Some readers may now be feeling a range of emotions from sadness to outright anger. People who have been victims of their own misunderstanding, encouraged by those who benefit, will react emotionally when they see what has been happening. The least feeling may be the emptiness that is left when a bubble bursts; you can no longer believe in the slimming ethic of calories and scales which once dictated your actions, and perhaps dominated your life.

The diet ingredients which seemed like a bad joke in Chapter 2 have turned up as the main constituents of the best-selling diets we have looked at. And none of them offers success in the long term battle against fat.

Diets like these make you fat because they all demand an imbalanced way of life. They vary in the degree of impossibility, but all involve dedication to perpetual fruitless (or, in some cases, fruit *ad nauseam*) suffering.

Dieting is *not* the way to be thin. If the metabolic shock which causes that initial loss of weight is initiated by food restriction, a predictable chain of events will be set in motion. The body will prepare for famine and conserve fat, and the metabolic rate will be depressed. This sequence can be very bad for health. Beauty is one aim of weight loss, but this is not the way to be beautiful; unhealthy people rarely look beautiful. In so many ways dieting is bad for many aspects of your *self*.

The apparent success of the diet shock leads to the trap of the diet seesaw. Daily food and nutrition disruptions become amplified over time, turning into the macro swings in body weight over a period of months or years which are typical of most dieters' personal histories. As the diet seesaw takes your weight up and down, the proportion of fat on your body increases, although you may weigh less. And tragically there seems no way to get out of the trap and off the seesaw, except perhaps the next diet . . .

The best dieters can hope for is to hold the seesaw down. The soul-destroying effort of this unending task produces a typical gaunt fragility; after years of battle the 'successful' dieter is characterised by haggard facial features and a thin, bitter look. It is a life with no energy, no *joie de vivre*, decreased resistance to infections and increased susceptibility to long-term disease and degeneration. Success for dieters is a miserable way of being half alive.

Why do people persist with such an unrewarding way of life? Dieters are trapped, the trap sprung by a distorted perspective of self which at times amounts to a pathological self-hatred. It is closed by an absolute lack of understanding of how to live with food. The obsessive calorie counting, which has now extended to cover the equally pointless counting of protein, fat, carbohydrate, sodium and cholesterol, is no substitute for understanding the crucial and ever-changing relationship between your self and your food. People who count consumption in this way are like the child who takes the clock apart looking for the tick; the more they search, the less they find. So the diet trap itself becomes a crucial part of the bigger fat trap: a part of the problem, not a way out.

Perpetual dieters are victims of distorted relationships, both with themselves and with food. To break out of the diet trap, to be thin if that is your desire, you need to accept your self, to be master of your food – and enjoy it! Then it will be possible to become the sort of person you are capable of being by working *with* your body, rather than continually fighting a losing battle *against* it.

The crucial key is within *you*. How you see yourself and how you direct your lifestyle are fundamental to success.

You cannot avoid this responsibility by following someone else's arbitrary and, at times, ridiculous rules. Nor can you replace understanding of your personal food needs with packets of standard chemical soups.

Success begins with a realistic understanding of what makes you fat. You have to forget the calorie myth. Explore yourself and your relationship with fat, and then change that relationship to your own advantage. It is as simple and as complex as that, and the next part of the book will guide your self-exploration.

Success will be complete when you are finally clear of the fat trap. Most dieters fail time and time again for one reason: no matter how thin they actually become through dieting and suffering, *they never stop thinking and behaving like fat people.*

Indeed it is an essential part of the diet trap that they continue to think fat; self-discipline and rigid denial are *not* characteristic of the thin people that fat people envy. No thin person is driven to frantic despair by gaining 2 lb (1k) of body weight as fat people are; they generally don't give a damn, because they know it will go just as casually as it came. The thin person has life, more or less, in balance; the fat person is still trying to hold that seesaw down.

While you think like a fat person, constantly obsessed by weight, diet, calories, scales and all the rest, you will remain a fat person. You *may* have periods of thinness, but fat will haunt you forever.

If you want to be thin, you have to think and live like a thin person. The first step is to say, loud, clear, and with conviction, 'Dieting be damned!'

PART II

Natural Slenderness

CHAPTER 10

What's Making *You* Fat?

If you understand what is making you fat, you can concentrate on whatever is necessary to be thin. This is so obvious it may seem silly to state it, but precisely what is making *you* fat may be far from obvious.

The majority of slimmers have one simple idea about what is making them fat: they believe they are eating too much. But as we have explained, simply eating less is usually not the answer; in fact eating too little can persuade the body to conserve fat.

A decade or so ago the idea that inactivity was an important factor was added to eating too much. If you wanted to lose weight you had to eat less and be more active. Aerobics, dancercise, jogging and all the other forms of increased activity were added to the armoury in the pursuit of slenderness. Yet many still found, despite the trials of hunger and exertion, that they remained fat.

Some people have come to the conclusion that for them fat loss is impossible. They have followed diets conscientiously, they have exercised regularly, sometimes to excess, yet fat clings to their bodies. Distressingly, some find that they can be slim except for lumps of fat which illogically persist on their belly or thighs, or in the form of localised patches of cellulite.

A minority may suspect that they are just destined to be fat. To this unfortunate few it seems at times as if they have only to breathe to put on more inches. Of course, that can't be true, can it?

As you have been reading this chapter you will probably

have reached a point of doubt. Perhaps you can lose weight by dieting, and keep it off to be vital and healthy. Perhaps careful eating and exercise work for you. On the other hand you may have found a point of recognition, perhaps in the failure of yet another diet, more likely in the impossibility of maintaining food restriction and exercise schedules. Increasing numbers of dieters will recognise the phenomenon of losing much but not all of their excess fat, or of finding that fat stays on whatever they do. Those who recognise a point of failure will far outnumber those fortunate few whose success enables them to cling to an old-fashioned understanding of fat.

Most people have an inadequate understanding of fat and its causes, and undoubtedly the majority of these would prefer to ignore it and hope it will go away; but it does not work like that. Understanding will allow you to direct your efforts so that they are effective, rather than just go through a ritual and hope it will work. We have to come to terms with fat, and in doing so we become better equipped to deal with it.

What do we need to know about fat?

First, we need to discard the idea that it is just passive storage for excess food. Second, we must realise that, when it comes to fat, men and women have very different bodies and metabolisms. Our culture makes many assumptions about the difference between the sexes in humans, and on the whole these are unhelpful in our understanding of fat.

We are all aware of the obvious sexual differences between men and women; after all, they are intended to be obvious. And we may be aware of the immediate implications of these differences, in terms of different hormones, body structure and behaviour. But the differences go much deeper. They are reflected in the way our bodies are fuelled, which in turn reflects the different ways we are intended to operate.

These differences arise because of the way we evolved over millions of years. Briefly it amounts to this: men developed high-level short-term endurance; they could hunt all day, and still sprint for the kill. After this, or an analogous situation, as every woman knows, men tend to gorge themselves and fall asleep. Women are designed for the long haul; they can work steadily for a long time, but their ability to produce a final sprint is limited. The characteristic endurance and persistence of women is something men may become familiar with.

These different activity profiles have produced different organic structures. Men have large livers which act as energy stores; the release of glycogen from the liver under the influence of adrenalin fuels that explosive burst of energy. They also have (or should have) less body fat to slow them down and large muscles which, as well as giving strength, act as primary energy stores. Women have relatively smaller livers and smaller muscles, but they have that thicker subcutaneous layer of body fat which provides long-term energy for feats of endurance which men could not cope with.

What are the practical implications of these differences? They mean that women should have a different eating pattern. This is why many women find family living and three meals a day very fattening. Women should nibble frequently, keeping their energy output and input in balance almost on an hour-to-hour basis – this is the essential truth of calorie counting. They should not have large meals followed by gaps – that is the male pattern essential to recharge glycogen stores. Regular meals are too big for women, and the gaps in between too long – that is the fallacy of calorie counting.

The other important implication of male/female differences also relates to the liver. Our livers are awe inspiring organs, nothing less than the industrial areas of our bodies. Together with the heart, the power station, the functions of the liver underwrite our very existence. One primary function is that of metabolising everything which comes into our body; while metabolic processes happen everywhere, it is the liver which is the central focus. The liver takes our food, in the form of digestion products, and reassembles it all into the substances we need for growth, repair and energy. The liver also deals with waste. The reason why women tend to get drunk easier than men is because their smaller livers cannot process so much waste, in this case alcohol. This is true of all the things the body has to metabolise; the female liver can become overloaded relatively easily.

If this happens with a substance your liver decides is toxic it has another trick in reserve. Instead of adding to its overload, or risking poisoning other parts of the body with breakdown products from metabolising the toxin, the liver will dump it in that convenient subcutaneous layer of fat.

If necessary, the liver will go further. If you have not got enough body fat for toxin storage it will ensure that fat is manufactured. So, no matter how well you control the calories, if your liver is overloaded with toxic substances, you could get fatter.

What do we mean by toxins? Classically a toxin is a poison. Today with millions of entirely man-made substances in every part of our environment, it may be anything which your body treats as poisonous. Here we confront the problem of individual variability in body response and weight loss. You may be able to live on processed foods in a chemically contaminated environment, smoking and drinking and happily metabolising all the substances that pass through your body. For your best friend, or even your sister, one whiff of the wrong chemical could cause her liver to start furiously ordering fat. Can breathing make you fat? Oh yes, in today's contaminated world it can, and much worse . . .

Fat is far from a passive food store, though most diet writers treat it in this way, and any attempt to treat it in this simplistic manner is bound to fail. Fat has a wide range of functions in our lives, from effects on reproduction to the molecular management of our metabolism. The amount we each carry will depend on the importance of fat's complex functions to each of us at various times in our lives, and these will vary as different circumstances affect us. To simplify the picture we can divide the functions of fat in women under four general headings:

1. Sexual attraction
2. Insulation
3. Food storage
4. Neutralising poisons.

Let us look at these in a little more detail. First, sexual attraction. It is very easy to overlook the fact that fat plays a large part in making women sexually attractive. The soft body contours and accentuation of breasts and buttocks are all formed by fat. It is the arrival of these deposits which signals sexual maturity in young females. It may be that resisting these changes, as the young girl is driven to maturity by forces out of her control, is at the root of much anorexia.

Second, fat acts as insulation. Under this heading we would include the subcutaneous storage layer, for although it is mainly intended as food, it probably evolved when we lost our fur and the more static females needed a little extra protection. The loss of fur also meant that pregnant females and their unborn children were more at risk from climatic fluctuations, particularly with those large and potentially chilly hip bones. Nature's response for sexually active females is to add a little extra to the reserves so that should she become pregnant, mother and baby will be warm and have energy reserves for survival.

Third, everyone knows that we store excess food as fat, and it is true that if our fat is attributable to excessive eating, eating less will make you thinner. The trouble is that few people's weight problem is that simple. If you are sexually active your body will be nudging your appetite; if the weather turns cold it will do the same; if your liver is overloaded it may do the same. If your eating is triggered by emotional stresses or social pressures, the additional burden of struggling to lose weight can add to the unhappiness that leads to eating – so that the harder you try to shed your fat, the more likely you are to over-eat. And of course you may just enjoy eating for many reasons unconnected with biological needs.

Fourth, fat provides protection against poisons. As we have seen, the conventional view of fat is that it is essentially passive, it is supposed to sit on the body, shaping by its position, insulating and storing energy. The fourth function of fat is an active one, that of a storage medium for substances the body treats as toxic. The body will tend to conserve this fat, and may at times generate more fat when it is confronted with an overload it can cope with in no other way.

With fat fulfilling all these functions in your body, many interacting pressures help to make you fat. Bear in mind that more than one different factor will be contributing to your problem; neither the problem nor its solution is one dimensional. You will probably find that you need to take action on many fronts at once. Many people find themselves apparently locked into their weight problem because they insist on trying to deal with only one aspect of its cause, usually by food restriction. But just as the various forces which make you fat interact with one another to potentiate the damage done by each, so action on many fronts to achieve a slimmer body and better health will make each aspect of the effort easier.

How do you know what is making you fat? How can you tell which approach you need to adopt to solve your fat problem?

Completing the questionnaire below will give you a good idea. You can then go on to the chapter indicated to further analyse and understand your personal fat problem. However, we would advise you to read all the chapters eventually, to be sure that you have taken account of all the factors involved.

If you are in any doubt, adopt the following priorities:

First, deal with your toxic fat problem. This will also correct dietary deficiencies.

Second, deal with any imbalanced eating.

Third, lose some insulation by improving your metabolism through healthy activity. This may involve eating more!

Lastly, do not try to remove that fat which your body needs to maintain its shape and resilience. Instead, concentrate on positive actions by improving muscle tone and proportions. Trying to become a skinny boy is a very dangerous thing for a woman to attempt.

What's Making You Fat?

The questionnaire below is designed to focus on the broad factors which are likely to be causing your weight problem. Choose the answer which is most true for you. If two answers fit you equally well, you can pick both.

1. What sort of food do you predominantly eat?
   a. A traditional diet of balanced meals.
   b. Wholefoods, organic if possible.
   c. Low-calorie 'diet' foods.
   d. Instant snacks and ready-prepared foods.

2. Do you suffer headaches or nausea after strenuous activity?
   a. Yes, often.
   b. No, I'm active but I don't have these problems.
   c. I do not have the energy for strenuous activity.
   d. Don't know.

3. Weight gain often happens suddenly after a particular experience. Did any of the following circumstances trigger your problem?

a. Illness or medication use (including starting the Pill).
b. Having a baby or starting to look after a dependent person.
c. Starting a new job, having the house done up or moving.
d. Loss of something or somebody that mattered to you.
e. Changing your eating pattern or food choices.

4. Look at yourself naked in a full-length mirror. Is your body
a. Rounded all over, generally in proportion?
b. Very big in the middle, with quite slim limbs?
c. Muscular but with large pads of fat on belly, buttocks, thighs?
d. You hate your body: it's disgusting.

5. Over the years, has your weight and size
a. Increased gradually but steadily?
b. Yo-yo'd wildly up, down, and up again?
c. Remained persistently high after a sudden jump from an acceptable level?
d. Increased stepwise to a series of successively higher plateaux?

6. Do you enjoy your food?
a. Not really; I feel guilty about eating it.
b. I adore food and everything concerned with it (except my fat!).
c. I tend not to think about food.
d. My choice of food is limited by allergies.

Interpreting your results

Your answers will fall into four categories, A, B, C and D, reflecting factors involved in weight problems. Count the number of answers in each column below to learn which factors are likely to be most important for you.

Factor	A	B	C	D
YOUR ANSWERS:				
Question 1	d	a	c	b
2	a	b	d	c
3	a or c	e	b	d
4	b	c	a	d
5	c	d	a	b
6	d	b	c	a

YOUR RESULTS

PREDOMINANTLY A
Your difficulty is likely to be due to problems with detoxi-fication. Substances that your body treats as toxic are stored in your fat and attempts to shed that fat flood your body with poisons. Your metabolic processes respond by locking your fat on your body to neutralise the toxins it contains. Read Chapter 11 to learn how to deal with toxic fat.

PREDOMINANTLY B
Your difficulty is likely to be with food: probably not so much over-eating as eating the wrong types of food. Read Chapter 12 to find out more.

PREDOMINANTLY C
Your activity level is not sufficient to keep your weight down. Find out how to burn excess fat more efficiently by reading Chapter 13.

PREDOMINANTLY D
Emotional problems trigger your weight gain. Learn more from Chapter 14.

CHAPTER 11

Persistent Fat:
Overcome the PFR Syndrome

Today everyone carries fat that is contaminated with artificial chemicals. A macabre anecdote often quoted to illus-
trate this fact is the American undertakers' discovery that
corpses stay unexpectedly fresh for weeks because of the
food preservatives they contain.

Every part of our environment is polluted with a great
variety of substances which can end up in our food and in
us. We take in many chemicals with everyday food, not
only acknowledged additives but also the residues of processing chemicals, pesticides and drugs. The air we breathe
and the water in our taps is contaminated with the waste
products of our industries, transport systems and daily lives.
Every one of the forty thousand or so artificial chemicals in
common use is to a greater or lesser degree a potential
metabolic hazard for some people. When our bodies treat
such substances as toxic, they may get dumped into fat.

In theory, this should be no more than a temporary
measure. The composition of our fat stores is continually
monitored, and when circumstances permit, the liver
should draw off the fat with its contaminants and deal with
them at a safe rate. Two problems may arise. First, if your
exposure to high levels of substances that your body treats
in this way continues, your liver will not have the spare
capacity required to process the toxins in your fat. Second,
your body may be loathe to process these toxins at all.
Having adopted the trick of fat production for toxin storage,
your metabolism may simply generate more fat whenever
you are exposed to chemical stress and lock that on rather

than deal with it. This produces the ill-proportioned mixture of fat and lean with which dieters end up.

If your metabolism decides to dump any substance into fat rather than deal fully with it, or to manufacture fat as a storage medium for such substances, persistent fat can result and you will confront continual difficulties when you try to shed that polluted fat. People whose bodies use fat in this way are victims of the Persistent Fat Retention (PFR) Syndrome. (A syndrome is a variety of effects caused by a general phenomenon – in this case, exposure to toxic substances.)

Because they do not involve a single specific cause and effect, syndromes can be particularly difficult to deal with. The PFR Syndrome is no exception. Understanding how the syndrome occurs can nevertheless enable individuals to get to grips with the problem and produce a solution that will work for them.

The defining characteristic of the PFR Syndrome is fat that will not shift. You may have fat on your body which you have been unable to shed through diet or exercise. Indeed, nothing seems to affect it, it is locked onto the body. The amount of persistent fat varies from person to person. Some unfortunate individuals are fat all over and deeply distressed by their condition. At the other extreme, persistent fat may form localised deposits which will not go away from thighs or arms. Many people experience it as cellulite or slabs of fat at particular body sites, most often on the stomach.

The causes of PFR fall into three general groups, all of which may affect susceptible individuals. These are:

1. Drugs, including both prescription and over-the-counter medicines, and substances used as recreational drugs.
2. Anything which triggers allergic reactions.
3. General environmental pollution.

That drugs can make you fat, despite their negligible calorie content, may come as a surprise. But weight gain is an acknowledged side-effect of hundreds of widely used medicines, from the contraceptive pill to drugs used to treat depression. Many recreational drugs, including alcohol and cannabis, can also lead to fat deposition.

Allergic reactions are part of a more complex problem and symptoms of overload in the immune system. In an allergic reaction, the body misidentifies harmless substances as toxins, which then add to the load on the liver. Whether caused by chemicals or natural substances, allergic reactions can increase demand for food input and slow the body down to facilitate dumping of unwanted substances into fat.

General environmental pollution is a catch-all term which includes any of the uncounted artificial substances released into the environment via the chemical and petro-chemical industry. These substances and their breakdown products end up in and on our bodies. They are in the air we breathe and the liquids we drink; our food is contaminated by them.

Artificial substances are used in every area of life. Plastics and perfumes, food additives and drugs, paints and polishes, sprays and lubricants, are created in ever-growing quantities, to end up as environmental pollutants. With very few exceptions, everything we once made from natural substances is now treated in some way, at some stage, with artificial chemicals. Paradoxically, even the cleansers we use for our homes and clothes are nothing short of chemical pollutants.

How does the body decide whether a substance is safe or dangerous, and how to deal with it? The discrimination is controlled by the immune system, which, to protect us from poisons and infections, must assess every molecule that enters our bodies. It may be a virus, a particle of food, anything at all. Special mast cells with libraries of molecular records are positioned at strategic points all through our body. If they encounter a substance that is known and safe, nothing happens. If it is recognised as foreign and dangerous, appropriate defensive action is taken. In extreme cases the mast cells commit suicide by degranulating and releasing a mixture of nasty chemicals to destroy the enemy. In allergies like hayfever, this action is inappropriate; but the chemicals, including histamine, cause sneezes and sniffles and make the sufferer miserable.

The immune system's actions produce debris which is carried to the liver for further processing, along with all the other substances that enter our bodies. The liver will normally recycle anything useful and consign the rest to waste. The first choice for waste disposal is to pass it out with water, and anything that is water-soluble is removed from the body in urine or sweat.

Disposing of fat-soluble waste is less straightforward. These wastes are dissolved in bile and carried back into the intestine to be excreted with solid waste. The liver has no direct output connections; waste is carried to the kidneys via the bloodstream and the heart, while, to further complicate matters, bile – whether contaminated or not – is recycled. Any chemical judged too dangerous for this leaky journey may be attached to a special carrier system to be dumped in fat. This may be the safest way to deal with it. But once your body has learned this response, it may use it more readily in the future, and it will not want to confront those chemicals when you try to lose weight. The result is persistent fat.

The truth is that pollution can make you fat. We are simply not designed to metabolise chemicals in such quantities.

The situation may not be as hopeless as it seems. If this is the cause of your weight problem, you have to persuade your system to deal more effectively with the substances it is treating as toxic. In effect you have to refine your fat; then you will be able to shed it.

The first step is to stop adding to the loading you are

putting on your metabolic processes. To do this, you have to identify the substances that represent particular problems for your body, and avoid them.

The questionnaire below will indicate the degree to which you may be susceptible to the PFR Syndrome, and suggest possible causes.

1. Do you suffer from asthma, eczema, severe hay fever or other allergies?
   Yes, I have very severe allergy problems: Score 6
   I have chronic allergy problems: Score 4
   I suffer some allergic reactions, but not always or not
   *   severely: score 2*
   Not at all: score 0

2. Do you use medicines (other than Cromoglycate or Intal) to control your allergies?
   Yes, regularly: Score 4
   Yes, sometimes: score 2
   Not at all: score 0

3. Are you sensitive to any common foods?
   Yes, many: Score 4
   Some, sometimes, or not severely: score 2
   Not at all: score 0

4. Do you react badly to solvents and fumes (eg glue, paints, smoke, fumes at work, DIY chemicals)?
   Yes, many of these: Score 4
   Some, sometimes, or not severely: score 2
   Not at all: score 0

5. Do you suffer from abdominal discomfort and diarrhoea?
   Yes, frequently: Score 4
   Sometimes, not severely: score 2
   Very rarely: score 0

6. Can you drink as much alcohol without illness as your friends?
   Yes, no problems here: Score 0
   I am more sensitive to alcohol than most people: Score 2
   I get very ill with quite small quantities: Score 4

7. Have you ever suffered from jaundice or liver disease?
   Yes, within the past 2 years: Score 4
   Yes, more than 2 years ago: Score 2
   Not at all: score 0

8. Do you suffer from nausea?
   Yes, frequently: Score 4
   Sometimes: score 2
   Rarely: score 0

9. Do you suffer from arthritis or frequent joint pains?
   Yes, badly: Score 4
   Sometimes, or not severely: score 2
   Not at all: score 0

10. Does excess fat accumulate particularly around your waist?
    Yes, my waist/tummy is very big in relation to the rest of my body: Score 4
    Yes, but I also put on fat all over: Score 2
    My proportions remain fairly constant when I get fat: Score 0

11. Can you relate the *onset* of your weight problem to any of the following: a course of medication; use of oral contraceptives; exposure to high levels of air pollution, fumes or pesticide sprays?
    Yes, definitely; no previous weight problem: Score 4
    More than one of these caused fat deposition: Score 6
    No clear link with any of these: Score 0

12. How does a session of intensive exercise make you feel?

    I suffer a severe hangover next day: Score 4
    Exercise quickly causes nausea and headaches: Score 4
    Both of the above: Score 8
    Effects of exercise vary; sometimes I feel ill, sometimes refreshed: Score 2
    Although tiring, exercise does not make me ill: Score 0

13. Are you: a) Below average height for your sex; b) Female; c) Both of these?

    a) Score 2; b) Score 4; c) Score 6

Add your scores together to assess your PFR problem.

INTERPRETING YOUR SCORE

Over 34
You have considerable difficulty dealing with many different substances; this makes you particularly vulnerable to persistent fat. Because your fat is playing an important protective role by storing those toxins out of harm's way, your body will try to retain it by reducing your energy levels very quickly if you try to lose weight by conventional methods.

Rapid weight loss could be very dangerous for you; dieting will probably induce raging hunger. If you persist in dieting, you are likely to become ill and your efforts will tend to have depressingly little of the desired effect. You are likely to find exercise unpleasant and difficult because it will release toxins from your fat as it is burnt by muscle action.

You should adopt the plan described below and not attempt to cut back your intake of food. Seek advice on specific allergy problems and try to pinpoint and avoid the worst offenders in your environment. A clinical ecologist or homeopath may be able to assist.

20–34

The PFR Syndrome contributes to your weight problem and you should be careful to avoid stressing your detoxifying systems when you lose weight. The toxins released into your bloodstream when you shed fat will limit your ability to do so safely.

If you keep conscientiously to a pure food diet (Chapter 12), avoid toxic stress and build up your liver capacity as we explain below, you will find that you will be able to lose unwanted fat much more quickly and easily. However, the process may take a year or more, and you must be patient. When you are no longer suffering the chronic mild poisoning which adds to your weight problems, you will feel very much fitter and have more energy.

8–20

While you do not seem to react badly to a wide range of substances in your everyday environment, problems with dealing with toxic substances hamper your efforts at weight loss. Awareness of this potential hazard and taking the steps described in this chapter should prevent it from becoming any worse. If you suffer limited or seasonal allergies such as hay fever, but are otherwise free of problems of this type, you can build your tolerance to your allergen by a combination of strategies such as we describe in our book, *Hay Fever – No Need to Suffer*.

Reducing your susceptibility to allergic and toxic reactions will help combat your weight problem. However, this is likely to be a relatively minor contributing factor and you should give priority to those areas of your life where your difficulties are greater. Remember that the effects of these changes are complementary.

Less than 8

Your body's detoxifying capacity seems to be quite efficient, although it may not always be quite sufficient to meet the demands of our polluted environment. Maintain your level of liver function through good diet (Chapter 12), adequate activity (Chapter 13) and avoiding over-indulgence in alcohol.

Drug Use

1. Do you regularly take any prescribed or recreational drugs?
   Yes: read (i) below.

2. How many measures of alcoholic drink do you have each week? (Check your four-day food and drink diary (see Chapter 12). Count as one measure ½ pint beer or cider, glass of wine, single sherry, single whisky or other spirit, or equivalent.)
   Women: 6 or more measures per week and
   Men: 10 or more measures per week: read (ii) below

(i) The following types of drugs are particularly often associated with weight problems:
   Sex hormones (including Hormone Replacement
      Therapy, the Pill, progestogens such as Duphaston)
   Steroids
   Antidepressants
   Tranquillisers

If you are taking any of these preparations, you can learn how to reduce your need for them by reading our book *Alternatives to Drugs*.

(ii) Alcohol contributes to weight problems in many ways. It is an instant energy source which can be converted into fat in much the same way as sugar; it damages the liver and interferes with detoxification; it usually contains a variety of other poisons such as sulphites which add to your toxin loading and which are often more difficult for

your body to handle than the alcohol itself; it can make you reckless, so that you eat types of food that you would normally avoid; and it interacts with other poisons such as those in tobacco smoke, potentiating their effects.
Anything more than occasional, low-level drinking is likely to be an important contributor to weight problems.

Women: 6–20 measures per week; men: 10–30 measures per week
You are a casual social drinker. Even this level of alcohol use will tend to add to weight problems; choose non-alcoholic drinks such as mineral water or diluted fruit juice more often.

Women: over 20 measures per week; men: over 30 measures per week
It is common knowledge that alcohol makes you fat; you have a weight problem, yet you continue to drink. Why? Heavier drinking usually reflects emotional problems, and you should try to deal with these at the same time as cutting back on the booze. If you try to stop drinking without dealing with the cause of your drinking, your efforts are not likely to be successful. See Chapter 14 for more advice.

The plan for dealing with persistent fat is this:

1. Avoid further contamination
2. Refine the toxins out of your body
3. Increase your metabolic capacity
4. Eliminate the unwanted fat.

There are some things you *must not* do if you suffer from the PFR Syndrome.
You must not:
Go hungry. This will only increase your PFR problem.

Overload your liver with drink, drugs or exposure to chemicals.

Attempt extremes of activity.

Let us work through the plan for dealing with PFR. Many people will not have to go all the way. For some, avoiding contamination may be enough, but most will have to alter eating habits as well, since these may be the source of contamination and changing eating habits will help to solve the problem. Work through the plan and allow your body plenty of time at each stage. With PFR you must make haste slowly.

1) Avoid Further Contamination

If you think the source of your problem is drugs, you may have to manage without, or at least reduce the quantity you take, before you can lose weight. You should discuss this with your doctor, and you may find our book *Alternatives to Drugs* helpful. But bear in mind that the fat you are carrying may have been caused by drugs taken some time ago. The complaint you took them for may have long gone, and left you with the fat.

Allergic reactions require a multi-faceted approach. You should first try to identify what triggers your allergy and reduce your exposure to it. With food allergies this usually means not eating the food; the challenge is to discover the particular foods to which you are sensitive. The most common allergy triggers are eggs, cows' milk and dairy produce, wheat and pork. Food colours and other additives are also common allergy triggers and you should avoid all additives except natural products such as E160 (vitamin A derivatives). Check one of the guides to food additives such as Maurice Hanssen's *E for Additives* for information on which are most likely to cause allergic reactions.

Respiratory allergies such as asthma are made worse by any form of air pollution, so avoid cigarette smoke and pay special attention to the issue of air pollution, discussed further below. Reduce your exposure to house dust mite by keeping your bedroom and bedding very clean. For those with hay fever our book *Hay Fever – No Need to Suffer* offers answers which will not make you fat but, remember, it is the allergic reaction itself which is the cause of the fat problem. You have to stop your body reacting, not cover up or mask the reaction. A good diet and regular exercise will help to reduce your allergic susceptibility, so read chapters 12 and 13 carefully. This applies to all forms of allergic reaction.

General environmental pollutants: try to reduce your exposure to all of these, especially any that you know make you feel unwell. Start by ensuring that you enjoy clean air. This is particularly important because the body has virtually no defences against toxins that we take in as we breathe. We did not evolve in a world in which air pollution was a problem. Chemicals move straight from the lining of our lungs into the blood stream. So . . .

Give up smoking and avoid smoke-filled rooms. Try to keep away from heavily polluted streets, traffic jams and busy cities during rush hours. Give up using sprays, 'air fresheners' and similar products. Household insecticides, timber treatments and DIY chemicals are particularly likely to cause problems: avoid them all. Never burn anything that produces foul-smelling smoke, especially plastics.

Fresh air is your ally against persistent fat. Your body needs oxygen to cope with toxins. Spend as much time as you can in the open air, breathing slowly and deeply.

There is no short cut in dealing with either environmental hazards or persistent fat. Patience and perseverence are the necessary virtues.

2) Refine the Toxins out of Your Body

To do this you must eat and drink only the purest possible things. In the modern world very little food and drink is uncontaminated. Fortunately a growing realisation of this, and of the deleterious effect of polluted food on health in general, is ensuring that alternatives are becoming more easily available.

You should aim to eat unprocessed organic foods (see Chapter 12). Drink pure fruit juices and bottled or purified water. Avoid tea, coffee, soft drinks and alcohol.

Specific foods of positive benefit for enhancing your detoxifying capacity include the following:

Fresh fruit rich in vitamins A, C and E. Good sources include all berry fruits, citrus fruit, melon and mangoes. Go for fruit with pink or yellow flesh.

Vegetables rich in iron and folic acid. All green leafy vegetables are good, especially if eaten raw. Grow your own beansprouts for the purest, freshest and most nutritious salads.

Nuts – particularly brazils, cashews and sunflower seeds – and free-range eggs. These contain important trace nutrients and amino acids essential to good liver function. Organic meat (especially liver) is excellent, but never eat liver from factory-farmed animals because the toxins to which they were exposed will be concentrated in the liver.

Make sure you eat plenty of the foods on this list every day. For a period of weeks, try to take things relatively easy to allow your system to get used to the new good food inputs. Do not stress yourself with demanding activity but take a daily brisk walk outdoors, breathing deeply.

Do *not* worry about your weight. You are refining the *quality* of your flesh. We will deal with the *quantity* later! Treat this period as one of good old-fashioned convalescence. Get enough sleep. Learn to relax completely. Stress hormones will add to the load on your liver and can contribute to persistent fat problems.

If you are a smoker – now is the time to give up! Yes, you may put on some weight (nowhere near as much as you would on a contaminated diet), but you will not lose your persistent fat if you smoke. The enzyme induction in the liver which smoking causes can help keep weight off but it also prevents the metabolism of toxic fat. You have to risk putting a little on in the short term so that you can lose a lot in the long run.

3) Increase Your Metabolic Capacity

The objective of this part of the plan is to help the smaller female liver become more efficient at dealing with toxins. There is only one way to do this: carefully designed activity with complementary eating.

Warning: If activity produces any sort of hangover effect afterwards, STOP. Exercise hangovers are caused by your body releasing toxins into the blood stream in excessive quantities. They will just be dumped back into fat, and may be more difficult to get into circulation next time.

If you suffer such a hangover, rest for at least three days, then try a lower level of activity. The object is to build capacity and mobilise toxins in quantities that you can cope with, not to overwhelm the body. Patience and perseverence.

If exercise hangovers continue, or you cannot face an increase in activity, you need a more specialised approach to PFR. Our book, *Persistent Fat and How to Lose It*, deals exhaustively with this problem and its solution. Remember you must deal with persistent fat before you can success-fully create the slim and shapely body you desire.

For those who can cope without such specialised help, the first phase of activity should be gentle and general. Even if you are not used to doing anything, the Canadian Air Force system described in *Physical Fitness* will be very useful. It is a graduated system which allows you to start very gently and build up as your ability improves. Be prepared to stick with it for some time. You have to get yourself fit to go onto the final phase of this part of the plan.

Second Warning: If you are over forty years old, and/or *very* overweight, you should be prepared to spend a long time on this phase. Little but often is the key.

For those who are reasonably fit and not too overweight, the next step is to increase metabolic capacity. To do this you should aim for the following. At least two, but not more than four, times a week you need to be able to indulge (oh yes, you should be enjoying it by now!) in a vigorous activity which keeps you sweating for at least half an hour.

This activity should be complemented by the following eating pattern: have a good meal two hours or more before your activity. Ideally your activity should take place in the evening, so that afterwards you can bath or shower and relax before going to bed. Drink as much as you need to make up the water loss, but try not to eat unless hunger is keeping you awake. Take it easy on your off days, and follow the eating pattern suggested in the next chapter.

After your activity, which should have caused your liver to discharge its glycogen stores, there will be a flurry of metabolic activity which will go on for up to 72 hours afterwards. Your liver will be recharging and increasing its capacity. It will be metabolising some fat and dealing with the toxins in it. It will also be rebuilding and recharging the muscular tissue you have been working, and clearing up the general debris caused by activity. Your heart will have been exerting itself during your activity, and it will continue to power all this activity by the liver. So take it easy, listen to your body, feed it if that is what it needs, rest it ready for the next session.

Final Warning: While your body is metabolising the toxins in fat you may have outbreaks of spots. Do not panic – spots are yet another method the body uses to get rid of things it does not want. In this case it is your immune system throwing out debris. Make sure you are eating enough good food to help the process along.

Over time a new physically competent you, with a firm

healthy figure will emerge. You may have some more fat to lose, but don't worry. Once you have solved your PFR problem the rest is easy. You can now locate yourself in Chapter 13 and go on from there.

Now you know what was behind your fat problem, and understand the total inadequacy of the advice offered by all those calorie-counting diets, you may be feeling angry about the lost years and effort. Don't waste your time and energy. You should be thinking about the state of a world where you, and millions like you, are made fat by the pollution in our environment.

Most of the junk that pollutes and affects us in this way is unnecessary, but highly profitable for the businesses which produce it. You have been a victim of the misguided view business and politics take of the global environment. Next time you hear Greenpeace or Friends of the Earth protesting or warning, listen. You have been affected by one of the things they have been campaigning about. This time your fat, by acting as a protective mechanism, saved you. Next time the results of ever more pollution could be more serious.

CHAPTER 12

Nutrition for Lifetime Slenderness

Poor nutrition is a very common reason for getting fat. Dieters and non-dieters alike are frequently malnourished on the characteristically over-processed, chemically contaminated diet which is the normal fare of the average British person. Dieters, who have deprived themselves of food for long periods, are especially likely to suffer from deficiencies of trace minerals and vitamins. Such deficiencies interfere with the efficient function of the body, reducing energy and capacity to cope with toxic or waste substances. These effects can make you fat both indirectly by reducing metabolic rate, and directly by triggering fat deposition within the body.

While good nutrition will not necessarily make you lose weight, it makes it easier for your body to burn fat. If you eat well, you will find activity (the *only* route to a leaner body) more enjoyable and less tiring. By eating more good food and becoming more active, you will increase your metabolic rate, gradually reversing the damage that you may have caused by dieting.

Eating well to shed fat is a long-term strategy. It will keep you healthier for the rest of your life. It does not depend on your endurance or ability to withstand hunger: quite the opposite. You should eat as much as you need to satisfy your hunger, without restricting your intake to stay within artificial rules that dictate what you are permitted.

The eating habits of our fast-food culture are responsible for a load of illness. In Third World countries, the diseases of our culture – diabetes, heart disease, arthritis, cancers of the breast and bowel – follow in the wake of changes from traditional eating patterns towards the model set by American multinational companies. Where the hamburger'n'cola empire expands, illness spreads in its wake.

Today in Africa, South America, the Pacific islands, among the remaining Indian tribes and the Inuit, fat people abound where there were none before. These populations are not well-nourished; they are malnourished. They have substituted junk food and sugar for their native unprocessed diets; and they are suffering epidemics of the diseases we die from in Britain. Getting fat is one of the early effects of the unbalanced diet that is largely to blame for this disastrous situation.

So how far is your regular diet to blame for your weight problem? Work through the questionnaires below to find out.

Food Choices Questionnaire

List *everything* you eat and drink on four consecutive days (including one weekend day). Do not pick days when you are being especially 'good' or when your normal eating patterns are altered for any reason. Study your list and use it to answer the following questions.

PREFERENCE FOR SWEETNESS
1. How many cakes, pies, sweetened scones or biscuits did you have?
   (Score 1 for each biscuit or scone, 2 for plain cake or pastry, 4 for rich cake or pie)

2. How many chocolate bars, concentrated fruit bars, 'muesli' bars or other sweet snacks did you have? (Include 'diabetic' and 'sugar-free' sweets.)
   (Score 1 for each ounce/28g)

3. How often did you have a dessert (other than fresh fruit)? (Include fruit yoghurt, ice creams, etc.)
   (Score 2 for each)

4. How often did you use jam, honey, or other sweet spreads? (Include 'sugar-free' and 'high fruit' forms.)
   (Score 1 for each teaspoonful)

5. How often did you have sweetened breakfast cereal or add sweetener to your cereal?
   (Score 2 for each occasion)

6. How many sweet drinks did you have? (Include 'diet' colas and any drinks with sugar or synthetic sweeteners.)
   (Score 1 for each teaspoonful of sugar in tea or coffee, 3 for a soft drink)

Add together your scores to get your total Preference for Sweetness Score.

FAT INTAKE

7. How many savoury pies, pastries or puddings did you have?
   (Score 3 for each)

8. How many portions of chips did you have?
   (Score 2 for each)

9. How many meals or snacks included meat or meat products?
   (Score 2 for each)

10. How much cheese did you eat? (Include cooked cheese dishes.)
    (Score 1 for each ounce/28g)

11. How often did you eat snacks such as crisps, cheese-flavoured savouries, salted peanuts?
    (Score 1 for each small pack)

12. How often did you have butter or margarine on your vegetables?
    (Score 1 for each occasion)

Add up your total for this section for your Fat Score.

WHOLESOME FOOD CHOICES
13. How many fresh salads did you have?
    (Score 2 for each)

14. How often did you eat fish?
    (Score 2 for each occasion)

15. How often did you eat fresh cooked vegetables?
    (Include boiled or baked potatoes, not chips.)
    (Score 1 for each portion)

16. Do you habitually choose wholemeal bread?
    (Score 4 for Yes, always; 2 for Usually)

17. Do you habitually choose wholemeal spaghetti, wholemeal pasta products, brown rice, other wholefoods?
    (score 4 for Yes, always; 2 for Usually)

18. Do you seek out organic food?
    (score 6 for Yes, always; 4 for Usually; 2 for Yes, but it's often impossible to find)

Add up your total for this section for your Wholesome Food Score.

FOOD CHOICES: INTERPRETING YOUR SCORES
First, add your Preference for Sweetness and Fat Scores together, then subtract your Wholesome Food Score. This will give you a

total Food Choice Score. Note that a pattern of good food choices will produce a negative score. For example, if Preference for Sweetness plus Fat Score came to 35 and your Wholesome Food score was 40, your Food Choice Score would be −5 because 35 minus 40 equals −5.

Read the section that applies to you below, then go on to pinpoint your problem.

FOOD CHOICE SCORE

Over 90: Very poor selection
Your food choices are important contributors to your weight problem. As time goes on, you are likely to suffer more and more unpleasant consequences of your style of eating. These could include heart disease, diabetes, bowel disease and cancers.

You know that you do not habitually pick healthy foods. Is this because you do not attach much importance to your diet? We can only reiterate the message that you must have heard many times before: good diet is crucial to good health. One way your body reacts to a poor diet is by accumulating fat. If you sincerely want to lose weight and stay slim, you need to change the way you eat.

This does not mean cutting out foods till you are left with a meagre pile of celery sticks and apples − far from it. It means selecting foods that help your body to function well, eating plenty of them. We give more information later in this chapter.

55–90: Poor food selection
You need to make radical changes to your diet. The reward of slimness and enhanced health does not actually demand significant deprivation − it just requires that you make the right choices and select foods that allow your body to function in the best possible way. Your problem is likely to

be with one particular group of foods, so read on to learn more.

20–55: Average selection

The problem with being average in relation to dietary choices is that the society into which you fit so neatly is an unhealthy one in which a great many people get fat. Those of us who tend to put on weight have to eat in an exceptional way in comparison with our culture – though the dietary choices that we must make are not so different from those of cultures where people stay slim and well into old age.

You probably already avoid foods that you associate with getting fat – but you may be avoiding things that you should be eating and you may not be eating enough of the types of food you need for enhanced health and energy. For example, are you substituting sweetened 'diet' foods for real nourishment? This is the sort of choice that leads to weight problems. Aim to eat more complex carbohydrate foods (bread, grains and vegetables) earlier in the day, so that you do not get hungry and fall victim to the temptation of less filling but more fattening types of food.

−15 to +20: A sensible selection

You know about diet and you take care to avoid foods that will tend to be harmful, while selecting wholefoods that will enhance your health. You could go further towards a healthy diet, and if you did, you would have greater success in your battle with the flab.

−15 or less: Excellent choices

Diet is not your problem – unless you binge on chocolate bars when you are not keeping a food diary! More on that below. Your pattern of food choices is generally good; are you eating as much as you need? While you make the choices you do, your only problem is likely to be that you get too little because of a mistaken belief that keeping yourself hungry is the way to shed excess weight. Don't fall into that trap! Your weight problem is not caused by the food choices you make now.

Now go back to your scores for the separate sections on sweetness and fat:

PREFERENCE FOR SWEETNESS
We focus on this aspect of diet because it is a particularly important cause of recurring weight problems. Whenever you eat something sweet, *whether or not it is high in calories*, your body reacts by producing a surge of insulin to deal with the anticipated sugar loading. This insulin production is *conditioned* to happen when you taste that sweetness. When your blood insulin level rises, sugar is removed from the blood and shifted into the tissues, where the insulin assists in storing it as fat.

Do not imagine that you are safe with synthetic sweeteners. Even when your sweet food or drink contains no sugar, your blood sugar still falls under the influence of insulin, and you will both lay down fat *and* feel hungry! Those 'diet' snacks and drinks that you probably thought you could have whenever you wished without increasing your fat problem are doubly bad for you.

Over 45
Your sweet tooth is a real problem. Even if you are substituting 'diet' products for the sugary foods and drinks that you love, you are causing problems for yourself. Until you cut down on these sweet foods, you will find your weight problem is very difficult to deal with. However, when you do learn to avoid them, you are likely to lose excess fat quickly.

The first step is always in your mind. You have to be determined that you will not go for sweetened food. That means refusing *all* sweetened foods, until you have unlearned your tendency to reach for them.

Many people find this easier than they expect. The key is to avoid getting hungry. Eat savoury foods earlier, and in larger quantities. Do not try to put off eating. Have some real food to eat when you might normally reach for a biscuit. What about a baked potato (with minted yoghurt, not butter!) at tea-time instead of cake? Or perhaps you'd enjoy a tomato sandwich? If you acknowledge your food needs and feed yourself properly, you will not be so tempted by things that make you fat.

Often the largest hurdle is killing the taste for sweet drinks. But even if you have always had sweetener in your tea or coffee, you will be surprised how quickly you can change over to the unsweetened form. Yes, it will taste horrible at first; you will need to be determined. Try taking your tea weaker if that's your stumbling-block. Or try a completely different hot drink, one which you have never drunk and therefore do not expect to taste sweet. A herb tea could be the answer. As for all those soft drinks . . . they are loaded with sugar! The 'diet' versions will swell your waistline too, as we have explained. Substitute *dilute* forms of natural fruit juice (such as sparkling apple juice) or mineral water such as Perrier.

Sour foods reduce your taste for sweetness. Cultivating a fondness for grapefruit will be very helpful – sweet food is simply horrible when you have that fresh grapefruit flavour in your mouth. Do not reject it after the first brief taste: let the juices remain in your mouth, where it will gradually come to taste sweeter as its enzymes change your perception of its flavour.

25–45

While you do not go overboard for sweet food or drink, it is contributing to your weight problem. Make cutting back an urgent priority. Read the suggestions we give above for those for whom sugar is a more serious matter and use this knowlege to reduce your dependence on sweetness.

Always read labels and reject foods with added sweeteners of any sort. Whenever you see a word ending in 'ose'
on an ingredients list, you are dealing with sugar; so reject
maltose, fructose, lactose and all other 'oses'. Sometimes it
will not be possible; lactose, for example, has many uses –
even as the carrier for homeopathic medicines; while sugars
such as fructose are not as damaging as ordinary sugar
(sucrose). But if you are conscious of the sugar problem
and your need to avoid it, you will find that your weight
becomes easier to manage.

8–25
Perhaps you do not think you need be any more concerned
than you are already about your intake of sweet food and
drink. Certainly, you take less than most people do. It
should not be too difficult to eliminate the remaining
sources of sweetness because you are not dependent on
them. Just remember our warning at the beginning of this
section: what it means, in a nutshell, is that sugar makes
you fat. And pseudo-sugar can make you fat too.

Sweet foods are fine for celebrations, special meals or
maybe once a week so that you do not feel unduly
deprived; but on a regular everyday basis – avoid them!

Under 8
Sugar is not your problem! Fine – keep it like that.

FAT INTAKE

Over 40
Do you really enjoy fatty foods that much, or do you just
accept what's convenient? Either way, with your fat consumption, it's no wonder you have a weight problem. You
would burn it all up if you worked as a lumberjack in the
snowy forests of the North – but you don't. So it is clogging
up your system and exposing you to a wide range of health

risks. High fat consumption is linked with heart and blood-vessel disease and cancers of the bowel, breast, ovaries and other organs.

Adding to the problem in our polluted world is the quality of the fat we eat. Many of the poisons produced in the developed world are fat-soluble, and animals store toxic substances in their fat. Most meats and meat products are high in fat, even if you can't actually see it. When you eat animal fat, you are exposing yourself to high doses of assorted toxins. Chapter 11 explains the consequences of this; in general terms, it will tend to make it harder for you to shed your unwanted fat, which will be polluted by the poisons in your food.

Cooked fat (especially fat that's kept hot or repeatedly reheated, like chip fat) carries its own risks. This oxidised fat is particularly difficult for your body to deal with. It is much more dangerous than pure, unheated fats such as cold-pressed oils. If you really want to eat fatty food, have it in the form of avocado or fresh nuts and seeds; in this form, it is nutritious and not dangerous.

Read on for suggestions on how to cut your fat intake.

25–40: average fat consumption
You are consuming far too much fat for optimum health and certainly too much for your waistline! Cut back by becoming conscious of the problem and choosing lower fat options whenever you can. That doesn't mean just substituting low-fat spread for butter – although you can do that if you wish. It means choosing baked potato rather than chips, and having low-fat yoghurt or cottage cheese on it, not butter or sour cream. It means choosing fish or fowl rather than meat. It means avoiding pastry products, especially pastry/meat savouries such as steak pies. If you need a snack, go for a salad sandwich (with the minimum of margarine or butter on the wholemeal bread, naturally!) Say no to meat and cheese more often – you probably eat

more protein than you need (most people do); instead, have more vegetable products.

8–25
While fat does not seem to be a major factor in your weight problem, you would benefit from cutting back on the fat sources mentioned in the questionnaire. Read the section above for specific advice on ways to achieve this.

Under 8
Your dietary choices in relation to fat seem to be excellent, and it is unlikely that your weight problem has anything to do with your fat intake . . . unless you are a secret cream fanatic!

SUGAR SENSITIVITY
1. Have you always had a sweet tooth?
    Yes, I adore sweet things!: Score 4
    I like sweets but resist them: Score 2
    No, I don't particularly prefer sweets: Score 0

2. Do you feel weak, tired, dozy or slightly crazy about an hour after eating a chocolate bar or sweets?
    Yes, but I can't resist them: Score 4
    Yes, and I avoid them: Score 2
    No, I have not noticed a reaction: Score 0

3. Do you feel dizzy, faint and irritable if you go without food for more than four hours?
    Yes, always: Score 4
    Sometimes: Score 2
    No, I just get hungry: Score 0

4. How much fruit do you eat each day?
    2 lb (1k) or more: Score 3
    1 to 2 lbs (½ to 1k): Score 2
    Less than 1 lb (½k): Score 0

5. Do you crave sweets, chocolate, or dried fruit?
   Yes, often: Score 3
   Sometimes: Score 1
   I don't get cravings for sweet things: Score 0

6. Do you suffer from diabetes?
   Yes: Score 10
   I am a borderline case: Score 8
   No, but I have been warned that I might: Score 4
   No: Score 0

Add up your total for this section for your Sugar Sensitivity Score.

INTERPRETING YOUR SUGAR SENSITIVITY SCORE
You should think about this score in conjunction with your Preference for Sweetness score, because the two are related. If you are highly sensitive to sugar, you will react more violently to it and it will be far more damaging to you. So if you have a lot of sweet food *and* a high score on this scale, cutting back your consumption of sweet food and drink is particularly important.

Over 18
You are very sensitive to sugar: beware! Avoid sweet things whenever you can; prevent sugar cravings by eating nutritious food in quantities sufficient to satisfy your appetite before you get too hungry and irrational. Because you react so strongly to fluctuations in blood sugar, it is especially important to keep it steady. A wholefood diet will help with this; oats and oat products (but *not* sweetened oat bars or biscuits), beans, peas and lentils, are particularly helpful. The fibre in unrefined wholefoods slows down the absorption of sugar and prevents both soaring blood sugar levels after meals and the rebound effect that follows insulin surges.

Insulin excess is the other face of sugar sensitivity. As

we have explained, insulin causes your cells to take up sugar. Reduce your insulin level by being physically active and keeping to a wholefood diet. This will make you feel better and more energetic while you solve your weight problem.

Excessive sugar sensitivity will cause an insulin surge in reaction to eating sweet fruit, although it will be less severe than that produced by processed sugar. Keep your consumption of fruit to about a pound a day. If you want more than this, it's probably because you are not eating enough starchy vegetables and grain products. Choose relatively sour fruit like grapefruit in preference to bananas, grapes and other sweet fruit. But if you cannot resist something really sweet, banana sandwiches or raisins are far better options than chocolate.

Reduce your sensitivity to sugar and insulin by adopting a more active lifestyle. If your activity score is low (see Chapter 13), your fat problem will be compounded. Attend to both at once, and you will be delighted by the results!

8–18
You do have a problem with sugar. Perhaps you have learnt from experience that sweet foods go straight to your fat stores and you know you cannot afford to eat them. If you are still eating sweet foods, you are putting your health at risk; you need to heed the warning signs and act decisively to protect yourself. See the section above for advice.

Under 8
You are not particularly sensitive to fluctuations in blood sugar so you do not have to be as rigorous in your avoidance of sweet foods as more sugar-sensitive people must be. This is probably because you have not been in the habit of overloading your body with sugar in the past. Don't start now!

Getting Your Eating Habits Right

To get slim and remain that way throughout your life, you need to establish eating habits that will create good health. It is not a question of adopting some extreme diet for a short while, then slipping back into your old pattern – the pattern that helped to make you fat in the first place. So start as you mean to go on, with a healthy and enjoyable diet that you can maintain indefinitely.

Below are the principles on which lifetime slim nutrition is based. For most of us, it is not possible to stick rigidly to all of them all of the time, we live in a far from perfect world; but you will feel the benefit of each change you make in the direction they indicate. And when this is your basic way of eating, the occasional lapse will not be a disaster.

You should:

1. Eat organic wholefoods
2. Cut down hard on processed and animal fats
3. Choose fish rather than meat
4. Eat more fresh (raw whenever possible) vegetables
5. Give up sugar and artificial sweeteners.

Let us expand on these principles.

EAT ORGANIC

A diet that will keep you fit and slim for life without hunger should be composed of nutrient-rich, minimally processed foods which are free from chemical contamination. This is the type of food that our bodies are intended to handle, and on which we function best.

If you eat only organically produced wholefoods you can get as close to this ideal as possible in our polluted world. We know that it can be difficult to get organic food in some parts of the country, but it is worth making the effort. Not only is it better for your health, it tastes better too. Older people know how flavourless today's produce tastes in comparison with what they ate in their youth. This is no illusion, the superior flavour of organic produce reflects its higher level of nutrients. By eating organic you treat yourself to the delicious flavour of real food that truly nourishes and satisfies your appetite.

Organic food may cost more. This is because it is not produced by highly subsidised chemical-based agro-business, and growing it requires more care and labour. You might consider that getting people back on the land and growing superior food to nourish the population makes more sense than polluting and poisoning to produce yet bigger EEC mountains of inedible surpluses. We hope when enough of us think this way the politicians will act so that *all* food is good for us.

By eating organically produced food you will be joining a growing movement which is working towards a new, healthy ecological balance on our land. Eating organic, as well as being good for you, is also good for all the other creatures which live on the land. When farmers poison or burn everything that is not the particular crop they produce, they kill the birds, the otters and the wildlife that survives in our fields and streams. No matter what the chemical farmers say, widespread use of pesticides kills off good and bad alike; in the end it produces dead soil which is washed away like sand in heavy rain. Chemical agriculture is making a green desert of our land.

Where can you find organic food? First try your local wholefood store; check the labels, if it is organic it will say so.

Your local market is well worth a visit. In many places growers come in once or twice a week with their own produce, and they will be happy to discuss their cultivation methods with you. Ask if they use pesticides and fungicides; ask about fertilisers: are they narrow chemicals or natural rich manures? Try to find someone who avoids all chemicals – but watch out for Eddie Grundy cowboys!

Some supermarkets now sell organic produce. Ask for it, and encourage your local supermarket to stock more.

Remember though, nature does not conform to a human view of perfection. Wholesome natural produce is often damaged by other creatures who also enjoy its quality. If there are greenflies on the lettuce, the odd caterpillar in the cabbage or a maggot in an apple, you should welcome it. Try looking on these humble creatures as the modern equivalent of the miner's canary. As long as the canary sang the men in the mine knew they were safe from poisonous gas. Where insects are happy on food, you are safe; where they are being poisoned, so are you.

Organically produced meat is not so easy to get, but it is becoming more plentiful. It is available from shops in some large cities, such as Wholefood in Paddington Street, London W1, and people like The Real Meat Company at East Hill Farm, Heytesbury, Warminster, Wiltshire (0985 404361) are expanding the supply.

The best source of information on shops which stock organic foods is *The New Organic Food Guide* by Alan Gear.

EAT WHOLEFOODS

Wholefoods are complete foods. That is, they are the complete nut, grain, fruit or whatever. Many people develop weight problems when they try to live on foods which have been processed to remove essential parts and improve manufacturers' profits. Profit is quite simply what food processing is all about; there is no other reason for doing it. Food processors and manufacturers have found that they can take natural food apart and sell all its components; you buy 'rice', but if it is white, the husk with its vitamins and fibre has been removed and sold elsewhere. Usually it is the most nutritious part which is removed, humans get what is left.

The resulting denatured and flavourless 'food' is then treated with flavouring chemicals, salt and sugar are added, it is enriched with fat, perhaps added calcium (from the milk lake), and fluffed up with air or pumped up with water, wholesomely packaged to appeal to the consumer, and sent off to the supermarket. There it can wait for a long time for someone to buy it because of the mix of chemical preservatives it is also likely to contain. This is the basis of our very profitable food industry, and our very fat and unhealthy nation.

Wholefoods are more satisfying, more nourishing, and if they are also organic, almost perfect. They provide the bulk we need for our digestive system to work properly, and they help keep blood sugar levels even. These factors are very important, and will work in your favour when fighting the flab. Always choose wholemeal bread and pasta, whole cereals like porridge oats, and brown rice rather than white. Most of these foods keep well, and can be bought in bulk to store if they are not easily available locally; visit your wholefood supplier and stock up with the best.

Eat wholefoods whenever you wish, whenever you are hungry. Use them for energy before activity; these bulky carbohydrates are necessary to burn fat, they will help you stay naturally slim.

CUT DOWN ON PROCESSED FATS
The average British diet packs a whopping 40 per cent of its energy value in fat – usually cheap saturated fats that make us fat without contributing any useful nutrients. Most slimming regimes limit the amount of fat permitted. But there is a danger in cutting back hard on all types of fat. You may not get all the trace elements you need.

The answer is to eat as little as possible of all fat contained in prepared foods. This means avoiding biscuits, pastries and similar high-fat products, as well as all fried foods. You should also spread your butter or margarine as thinly as possible and avoid high-fat sauces and ready-made salad dressings.

Unprocessed fats are a completely different matter. Cold-pressed oils, such as organic olive oil, form a valuable part of the diet, protecting you against common types of illness. So do not hesitate to use them in your salad dressing. Oil rich foods, such as nuts, seeds and avocados, are important sources of trace nutrients that many British diets lack. This is another example of the error simple calorie counting can generate – one fat calorie counts the same as any other but the fats are crucially different. Unprocessed vegetable fats and fish oils will help your metabolism work better. Raw sunflower seeds are a particularly versatile and valuable addition to the diet; we nibble them on long journeys, mix them in green salads and in muesli, and cook them in nut roasts.

CUT DOWN ON ANIMAL FATS

Just like humans, other animals concentrate toxins in their fat. Today all animal fat is polluted, so it is not a good idea to eat it. This pollution will add to your weight problem, making your fat stores more difficult to shift. Animals reared on organic farms without drugs are the best source of animal products, but even they are affected by the spread of chemical pollution throughout the environment.

Avoid animal fat products as much as possible. Use skimmed milk, and if you adore cheese go for the least polluted forms. Organic cheese is available (we like Cardigan), or pick low-fat sorts. British cheese is certainly not best; we have a much worse record on chemical pollution than the cheesemakers of Holland, Norway, France and New Zealand.

Free-range eggs are superior to every other sort, particularly 'farm fresh', which translated means industrialised battery produced eggs. Eat free-range eggs as often as you like; avoid all others.

CHOOSE FISH RATHER THAN MEAT

Vegetarians are, on average, 20 lb (9k) lighter than meat eaters. They are also healthier and live longer. Nobody can really be happy about meat, either the way it is 'produced' or the pollutants it carries. Is it time you said goodbye to your butcher?

Fish is the least polluted of the flesh foods, and would get better if the seas around our islands were cleaned up. The fats in fish like herring are particularly beneficial to health. So if you are not ready for a complete shift to vegetarianism, why not try a change to fish?

EAT MORE VEGETABLES

All vegetables will help you to keep slim. That includes potatoes and other starchy vegetables.

You should go for fresh vegetables, organically produced if possible. Try to avoid ready-packed frozen and tinned vegetables, which are chemically grown varieties, often with added nasties to make them look good. Tinned vegetables generally have fewer nutrients than frozen, but any vegetables are better than none. Read labels carefully to see what has been added and reject any that include sugar or colours.

Raw organic vegetables are by far the most nutritious. Try to have salad every day and nibble raw vegetable sticks (*crudités*); you could grow your own to ensure supplies. Forget the English apology for salad, that leaf of lettuce and half tomato; go for variety and make sure you eat *enough*.

Make your own simple salad dressings with cold-pressed oils, from good wholefood shops, mixed with organic cider vinegar. Or you could try natural yoghurt with chopped fresh mint or other herbal flavouring. Experiment, see what suits you best, after all, you are not on a *diet*, are you?

GIVE UP SUGAR

Pure white sugar is so far from being a nutritious food that even moulds won't grow on it. Leave it in the pantry, and the mice ignore it. They are quite right. The nutritionist John Yudkin summed sugar up in the title of his book, *Pure White, and Deadly*.

Sugar addiction is part of the fat/diet trap. You don't need it and you will be happier and healthier without it.

Eating Patterns

In Chapter 10 we explained how differences between male and female physiology indicated that men and women should adopt different eating patterns.

Women should eat many snacks or small meals throughout the day. They should never go hungry, and food input should take account of activity levels and the other factors which influence appetite. The aim is to keep input and output in balance as far as possible, so that none of the metabolic alarms and demands which lead to fat conservation are initiated.

For single women this need present no problem. Your boss will rapidly get used to you eating the odd sandwich during the day at work, and if you eat out in the evening you can spread eating with chat so that you are not taking on a great load of food at once.

Women who are endeavouring to break out of the PFR Syndrome (Chapter 11) are the exceptions. They need to eat more like men, with fewer, larger meals without snacks in between. Most men will recognise this pattern as the one that suits them best.

Family life can be very fattening for wives and mothers. Those men demanding set meals two or three times a day tend to form the focus of the daily routine, and this can provoke conflict. You may have to adopt a dual regime to match the dual demands of your household. Good snackable food for women should always be available, while men get the large meals.

Many women find that they are hungry at mid-morning and mid-afternoon, especially when the children return from school; they should have their extra meals at these times. By dinner time, women who have already eaten a couple of hours earlier are likely to want only to nibble; a plateful of vegetables with gravy or salad dressing will probably be quite enough.

This pattern is common among tribal people, where women and children eat what they call 'human food' – the fruits, nuts, eggs and vegetables which they gather – while men, the hunters, get stews of meat or fish and starchy vegetables with the local equivalent of bread. Women prepare the food and tidy up whatever is left at their leisure, after the men have eaten. We should aim for a modern version of this very successful method.

The right eating pattern and a diet of organic wholefoods, will ensure that your body is well nourished and not subject to pressures which initiate over-eating. When you have achieved this you will be well on the way to mastering food and flab.

CHAPTER 13

Build a Lean Body

If you were directed to this chapter by the questionnaire in Chapter 10, with an indication that inactivity is the reason you find it difficult to be slim, you are likely to be feeling one of three things. Either you will be reading with an emotion bordering on sullen resentment – not sweaty nastiness again, I hate it – or you will be protesting that you are, despite the questionnaire – which must be wrong – already active all day long, and could not possibly do more. And some will be muttering, it's all very well for you two authors to say this, but you don't know about all the problems/difficulties/injuries, etc . . .

Perhaps one in three readers will be here with an open mind. They may have found some pleasure in aerobics, running or some other sporting type of activity, or just have the inner knowledge that activity is the answer and hope for encouragement. It is our task to get all our readers to the point where they accept the idea that a lean figure, health and beauty are practically impossible without regular physical activity.

Do not think that if you are very old, very over size or even partially immobile, or any of the possible combinations of these, this does not apply to you. It does! Mobility and movement are essential keys to improving your situation; you may have to make more effort than those who are younger, lighter and more agile, but the same principles apply. The basic lesson of all body systems is that if you don't use it, you will lose it. This even applies to fat. If you don't use your fat as a toxin store, as protection against famine or as insulation, you will lose it. So everyone will benefit from some well directed effort. Don't worry about where you are now, the recommendations below allow for all ages, sizes and abilities.

Dieting is essentially a passive process. This may be a large part of its appeal. So long as the calories are held in check, demure dieters can pose in the wings of their imaginary version of *Dallas* or *Dynasty*, all dressed up and waiting to be slim enough to go somewhere. Passive dieting is as much an illusion as the rest of the fantasy. Those who want a slim body like Joan Collins, Jane Fonda or any other superstar, will have to come into contact with reality – just as the stars who weave the fantasies do in their real lives.

Humans are just like any other animals. If we are active we keep fit and healthy. If we are not active we become sluggish and fat, and suffer all the degeneration that inactivity brings. There is no way around this basic truth.

Let us compare the advantages of the active approach with the passive in various areas of concern to most people who want to be thin.

The primary objective of any slimmer is to produce a body which is not only slim but attractive. Although you may be focusing on what fat does to your shape, underneath are the muscles which determine your body shape. Physical activity produces well developed (not excessive) muscles, in good condition, which will give you the final shape you want. Passive dieters take pot luck. Younger people may be able to return for a while to what remains of the bloom of their youth; most find more of the pot than the luck in the results that passive dieting produces.

The implied value of being slim is that it will release that vibrant vital you that is smothered by excess weight. Passive dieting, with its metabolic suppression, imbalanced nutrition and simple undernourishment, produces exactly the opposite. The habitual dieter is characterised by weakness and lethargy. Activity and a well fuelled body produce vitality by making sure that reactions are sharp and muscles are full of energy. The mind of an active person has an inner confidence in ability; it is not bound and restricted by the obsessions of the dieter.

Activity ensures the best chance of life-long health, the indispensable foundation for fulfilment and beauty. Passivity produces a poser's facade, behind which degeneration and a deep lack of satisfaction continually increase. We talk to many people, both dieters and those involved in various activities and sports. One thing distinguishes the two groups. The active ones are much happier, much more likely to laugh and show enjoyment.

To sum up the case for activity and against passivity there is one overwhelming reason for activity. It is that thing which passive dieters desire above all, and fail to achieve. Active people tend to be much more *in control* – of their bodies and of their lives. Those who stick to the passive approach tend to remain victims, both of the apparent vagaries of their bodies and also of their lives.

We hope we have convinced you that activity is essential for a lean body. Let us now deal with some common blocks which may be preventing you from turning the idea into practice.

For people who have been eating processed food and depriving their bodies of adequate nourishment, activity will have been a very unpleasant experience. Your body will have objected, in all sorts of painful ways, to expending energy. You have been conditioning it to malnutrition and starvation, and it will have been desperately trying to conserve the meagre resources you have supplied. This is the very opposite of what activity demands. In effect, trying to be active under these conditions has been adding injury to insult. A well nourished body will thrive on activity, and you will find that instead of punishing you, your body will reward you.

Those slim people who are constantly active are rewarded, not only by being attractive, but by the chemical changes that regular strenuous activity produces in the brain. Moods can be dramatically altered for the better, pre-menstrual tension (PMT) and other hormone-related problems can be reduced, and rising confidence brings a totally new outlook on the world.

For those who are constantly busy, and have no time for more activity, the problem is slightly different. Their routine tends to be one of constant distraction without achievement. They are going through the motions without gaining any benefits. The constantly busy need to stop – and build more purpose into what they are doing.

For most women this sort of activity tends to be focused on others, on children, husband or wider family. It grows over time into increasing commitment to others. Much of it can be dumped without ruining the relationships involved; for instance many women continue servicing the needs of growing children when those children should be looking after themselves. The rewards of the role of wife and mother can have too high a cost; perhaps the time has come for you to be more selfish, to seek more direct rewards in your own life. Paradoxically, both you and your relationships will benefit from a more fulfilled and independent you – although there is bound to be resistance to the change. Could your relationships be contributing to your inactivity and fat?

The other side of the activity equation is equally important. Purposeful physical activity *must* be balanced by adequate rest and recuperation. It is during these periods that the benefits are achieved; your metabolism re-orders and repairs your body, muscles are recharged with more energy, and the liver deals with toxins. Those subtle, desirable changes, stimulated by activity, occur during recuperation. Make sure you get enough good old fashioned relaxation and sleep.

If you are still looking for a way of copping out of becoming more active, you may have to go back to Chapter 9. Could your remaining objections, excuses and all the immovable blocks you are maintaining, exist because you are still thinking like a fat person? Try the attitude question-naire below to see if you are ready to go on.

Attitudes to Exercise

(Score 1 for Agree Completely; 2 for Agree Somewhat; 3 for Don't Know; 4 for Disagree Somewhat; 5 for Disagree Completely)

1. I have *never* enjoyed physical activity.
2. Exercise is no real help in weight loss.
3. I am too ungainly for sports.
4. I feel embarrassed in sports clothes.
5. Exercise would endanger my health.
6. I am too busy to find time for exercise.
7. I do not feel that I need exercise.

Add together the scores from all 7 questions to work out your Attitude to Exercise score.

INTERPRETING YOUR SCORE

Under 20
You resist suggestions that you should be more active. You may justify your attitude in a variety of ways, perhaps finding different reasons at different times for avoiding exercise. The outcome is always the same: you don't take it up, and if you do decide to try it your efforts are half-hearted and you give up very easily.

Before you can come to grips with your weight problem, you are going to have to work through your negative attitudes to exercise. Try to pinpoint their source.

Did your mother stop you playing active games for fear you might get hurt or dirty? Did you grow up in an inactive household where strength was seen as unfeminine or you learnt that brawn and brains didn't go together? Did enforced activity at school, where you always came in among the last stragglers in the race and never played anything well enough to be in one of the teams, turn you off exercise? Does exercise conjure up an image of goose-pimply thighs on a windswept playing field or great hulking Amazons? All of these, or other early experiences, could have contributed to your avoidance of activity.

Remember that the types of activity you can create for yourself now will not have any of the unpleasant features that you may have experienced in the past. You are not going in for competitive sports where your inferior performance will be obvious and shameful. You are not going to punish yourself by going out in standard sports clothes and exercising in all weathers. You can choose your time and style of activity yourself, so that you get maximum enjoyment from it.

When you do get into activity, you will make a marvellous discovery – it is intensely pleasurable! You will feel more proud of yourself and more comfortable with yourself than you have done for a long time. And you will experience the relaxation and mild euphoria that comes with physical exertion.

Physically demanding activity has subtle effects on the chemistry of the brain which produces these remarkable benefits. It changes the levels of the neurotransmitters (the chemicals which carry nerve impulses) which determine mood and energy levels, giving a sense of alertness and well-being. If you begin an exercise session feeling tired and depressed, within quite a short time your mood will lift. You may suddenly see how you can solve a problem that had been bothering you, or just experience a welcome sense of freedom from worry. And when you have built regular exercise in your life, you will find that the physiological changes it induces will help you to sleep and function better in every way.

You may benefit from help from an experienced person to get over some of the mental barriers that prevent you from enjoying your physical self. Listen to your physically competent friends and learn from them. Try joining a gym or evening activity classes where you will get individual attention and instruction. Talk to the people there; find someone you can relax with, and explain your difficulties. As soon as you have overcome those barriers, you will find a whole new universe of enjoyable experience – and an answer to your weight problem.

20–28
You are doubtful about the value of exercise and reluctant to do enough. The answer might be to look harder for a type of activity that appeals to you. Do you want to spend more time alone, or with other people? Choosing an exercise routine that you can do on your own could allow you the privacy you may require. Alternatively, joining a group could improve your social life as well as your physique.

Perhaps you want to remain unnoticed until you feel your figure is more appropriate for a sportsperson. Fine, work out a routine that does allow you to be inconspicuous – just so long as you stick at it long enough for your embarrassment to dissipate! Bicycle riding and brisk walks could be your answer, alternating with indoor workouts at home. You don't have to put on shorts and jog down the road if you feel you would look silly – there are plenty of other ways to work your body.

Over 28
You do not have anything against activity in principle, and if you do less than you need to keep in shape, it is probably because you have not made it a sufficiently high priority. You may not have been eating enough good food to have the energy to enjoy exercise – but the next section should help with this. Exercise does demand time and determination but it produces benefits in proportion to the energy

you put in. You will work better, look better and get more pleasure out of life if you do take sufficient exercise.

Now you have sorted out your attitudes, you are ready to go on to the questionnaires that will point you towards the sort of activity pattern that you should adopt. There are two things you should bear in mind. The first is that exercise is itself a substitute for a naturally active way of life. Living in the city, where basic needs are met on tap, does not make the sort of physical demands on us that might, from a health point of view, be in our best interests. So it is necessary to appreciate that exercise or sport must become a natural and regular part of your way of life. It should be built in, not just adopted at intervals when you feel you've got out of shape.

The second point is that although you may find it difficult at first, you will find it very easy to maintain your desired state once you have tuned yourself up and lost that unwanted fat. Chapter 15 tells you how.

Get yourself equipped. The minimum needs are good training shoes, cotton sports socks, a track suit and a cotton vest. These are as essential for health in the modern world as your toothbrush.

The next two questionnaires are designed to assess first, your physical capability now; and second, how active you actually are. Go through them both, noting the numbers of specific advice sections to which you are referred, and which you will find at the end of the questionnaire interpretation. Work through them in reverse order, that is, high numbers first.

Warning: If you are in any doubt about undertaking any sort of activity, or if you are on long-term medication, discuss your plans with your doctor.

CURRENT PHYSICAL CAPABILITY

1. How old are you?
   Under 33: Score 0

33–44: Score 1
45–59: Score 2
60–69: Score 4
Over 70: Score 6

2. Pinch a fold of loose flesh at your side, just below your waistline. Estimate the thickness of the skinfold between your finger and thumb.
   Less than 1" (2cm): Score 0
   1"–2" (2–5cm): Score 1
   2"–3" (5–7cm): Score 2
   Over 3" (7cm): Score 4

3. Compare your current weight with your weight at the age of 20. (If your weight fluctuated, use the weight you maintained for the most time at that age, not the maximum or minimum.)
   Within 10% (about 1 stone/6kg) of your weight at 20:
   *   Score 0*
   10–25% above weight at 20: Score 1
   25–40% above weight at 20: Score 2
   40–65% above weight at 20: Score 3
   More than 65% above weight at 20: Score 4

4. Do you have any health problems (eg heart problems or arthritis in knees or hips) which significantly reduce your mobility?
   Yes, walking is very difficult or impossible: Score 10
   My mobility is severely impaired, though I can walk: Score 9
   My mobility is restricted by health problems: Score 8
   Strenuous activity is impossible for me: Score 6
   My health problems make exercise difficult: Score 4
   I do not have health problems of this type: Score 0

Add your scores from each question to get a total Physical Capability Score.

Over 20

Your combination of overweight, health problems and age makes activity difficult. You must not allow this to prevent you from taking any exercise at all because a higher level of activity will improve your health, reducing the risk of cardiovascular disease and cutting down any pain you may suffer. Even if you are in a wheelchair, you can use your upper body – and it is very important that you do so. Get inspiration from disabled sportspeople; remember that people in wheelchairs regularly compete in marathons.

Swimming is one of the best forms of exercise for overweight or disabled people because it uses the whole body but does not stress the joints. Seek out a warm pool in your locality and join (or form) a group of people like yourself, in whose company you will be able to swim without embarrassment. If you are under treatment with a physiotherapist or other health professional, ask for advice about exercise that would be particularly suitable for you. There may be a therapeutic gym in your locality to which you can be referred.

Warning: Never take extra medication to prevent pain that you anticipate as a result of exercise. Always keep your level of activity well below that which could cause serious discomfort.

Refer to Sections 6, 9 and 10.

14–20

You have to be careful with exercise but you know you can do it and you should probably be doing more than you do at present. Do not be afraid of becoming more active: the benefits are much greater than the hazards. It is all too easy to convince yourself that activity is too difficult, you cannot do it; but this road leads directly to disability – your condition will deteriorate.

Start your exercise programme gently but make sure you stick to it even if it seems to produce no immediate benefits. This is a long-term strategy and essential for your health.

Refer to Sections 4, 5, 6 and 10, below.

Under 14

You can and should be physically active, and you are not likely to be at any particular risk – though everyone over about 40 and more than a couple of stone overweight should avoid strenuous exercise until they have become accustomed to putting this type of demand on their bodies. Always build up gradually to more intense activities and *never* 'go for the burn' or take up any physically punishing exercise schedule. Do not carry on in the face of pain – especially chest pain. It is a hazard warning that you should never ignore or try to override. Very sore or stiff muscles should be avoided as far as possible – they do not improve the rate at which you burn fat. If you do push yourself so that your muscles are stiff, give them time to recover completely before your next session of similar exercise.

Refer to Sections 3, 4, 5, 6 and 10, below.

Go on to the next questionnaire and learn whether you are active enough to be slim.

ARE YOU GETTING THERE?

1. How many miles do you walk outdoors each week?
   (Score 1 for each mile)

2. Measure 2 miles on level roads or paths using a map or car mileometer. Walk this route as fast as you can. How long did it take you? (Disabled people or those with health problems which prevent them from walking regularly should not attempt this.)
   Over 50 minutes, or task impossible: score 0
   40–50 minutes: score 3
   35–40 minutes: score 6
   30–35 minutes: score 10
   25–30 minutes: score 15
   less than 25 minutes: score 20

3. How many of the following did you do in the last week?
   (Score 5 for each occasion you spent the time given for each type of activity, 12 for each session of double length)

   a. Played an energetic game of tennis, squash, football or other sport (20 minutes).
   b. Swam vigorously (10 minutes).
   c. Ran continuously (10 minutes).
   d. Worked out on the floor (aerobic exercise or dance) (20 minutes).
   e. Cycled hard (20 minutes).
   f. Worked out with gym equipment or weights (10 minutes).
   g. Rowed hard (10 minutes).
   h. Climbed a steep hill or stairs (15 minutes).

4. How many of the following did you do in the last week?
   (Score 5 for each)

   a. Sawed or chopped logs by hand.
   b. Dug a garden or allotment.
   c. Mowed a lawn with unpowered mower.
   d. Rode a bicycle.
   e. Painted, plastered or built a wall.
   f. Did other similarly physically demanding work.

5. Do you wear high-heeled shoes on most days?
   (Yes: Subtract 10 from score. No: 0)

6. Do you have a pair of comfortable walking or running shoes?
   (Score 10 for good-quality training shoes
   Score 5 for comfortable walking shoes
   Subtract 10 for no sports shoes)

7. Are you rushing about all day at work or coping with your normal routine?
*(Yes, definitely: Score 10; Yes, usually: Score 5;
No, not really: 0)*

Make a note of your total: This is your Activity Score.

Over 100: Very active
You are fit and you enjoy using your body. Do you really have excess fat or are you trying to achieve a fashionable body shape that is far from that you were born with? The problem is more likely to lie in your *attitude* to yourself than in the form of your body. Stocky, muscular people can be lean and healthy but remain heavy because lean flesh weighs more than fat. Your body functions well; carry on using it as you do and it will look good well into old age.
Refer to Sections 1 and 2, below.

75–100: An active lifestyle
This is a good maintenance level of activity that should be sufficient to keep you lean. If stubborn fat persists, you may have reached a plateau where your body is no longer sufficiently stressed by your activity regime to change its composition. Try an activity that makes you work harder. For example, if you normally do aerobics three times a week, go running instead: running is the most effective way to burn fat fast. But do make sure you eat enough to support the extra effort!
    Read through the next section, noting particularly the points about anaerobic exercise.
Refer to Sections 1 and 3, below.

55–75: Moderately active
While your problem is not directly due to insufficient exercise, you would probably benefit from increasing your activity level.

You may need to put in more energy, rather than more time. If you are already jogging round the park, it could be time you rejected the idea that you should always have enough breath to chat; build in some hard running and sprinting. You may think you look ridiculous, limbs flying in all directions – we're not all naturals! But mixing demanding activity with less demanding activity enhances the effectiveness of your exercise tremendously. The body continues to burn fat for many hours after a session of *anaerobic* exercise (the sort that you cannot keep up for half an hour, that gets you panting really hard).

The most effective sort of exercise for weight loss alternates heavy demand (anaerobic) with longer-lasting, less demanding (aerobic) activity within each session. Ideally, a session should last a minimum of half an hour, because the body takes some time to start burning fat. Mixed walking, jogging, running and sprinting is perfect. Start gently, build up to a sprint, return to gentle activity, sprint again (or run uphill), wind down, and relax. We call it working through the gears. It's effective!

Refer to Sections 3 and 4, below.

40–55: Average activity level

Inadequate physical activity is likely to be one of the contributing factors for you. When your lifestyle is not sufficiently physically demanding, appetite and fat-turnover mechanisms do not operate as they should. You will want more food than you can use properly. This is one of the most important reasons for the gradual spread of weight problems throughout our society. With our cars and labour-saving devices, our normal level of activity is simply too low for most people to remain fit, slim and healthy.

Perhaps you have tried exercise and discovered that it is hard work and apparently ineffective; or perhaps you have been persuaded by all those diet authors that you cannot burn calories at a satisfactory rate through exercise, so you have lost whatever interest you might have had in it. Junk these ideas! Make a resolution to increase your regular activity level. If you fail to do so, you are not likely to become permanently slim.

Read the section below for advice on getting back in touch with your body so you can begin to enjoy exercise more. Then make a list of types of activity that you would like to take up on a regular basis, and set about building them into your life.

You may retort that you have no time or energy for exercise. Are you one of those who feels so worn out from constant dashing about that you imagine more activity is the last thing you need? If so, you are not taking enough time for yourself. Perhaps you think you do not really need time off, or can't afford it because there is always so much to do. You are wrong!

Slow down, review your life, consider your priorities. Write down all the things you have done today and yesterday and study your list critically.

Was all that rushing about actually necessary, or was much of it the product of your inability to say no to people who make inconsiderate demands on your time? Was it the product of guilt about being less than perfect? Was it a screen of empty activity that you built to hide behind? Are you expecting too much of yourself, undervaluing yourself, accepting the role of dogsbody or skivvy? Are you giving so much of your time and attention to your work or family that you have nothing left for yourself? This is a very common pattern among unselfish people, but in the long run it leads to serious health problems. We all need time for ourselves to unwind and assess our lives.

Activity and structured relaxation will start to build up positive feelings and increase the strength of your calm core. Your life will become less frenetic and more productive. It isn't just a question of using exercise to burn calories or tone muscles – activity can do far more for you. Use it! Refer to Sections 4, 5, 6 and 8, below.

20–40: Not sufficiently active
At this level of activity, a weight problem is very difficult to avoid. It is often accompanied by emotional problems such as nervous tension, depression, fears and phobias, and addiction to tranquillisers, including nicotine. Physical problems such as heart and circulatory disease follow as you get older. Increasing your level of physical activity will make you feel very much better as well as improving your appearance.

Imagine you are a child. Watch those skinny boys as they dash from place to place. That's how they stay skinny! But they love it, too. All that dashing about makes them feel much happier than they would if they moved slowly, ponderously.

If you're going shopping, go *as fast as you possibly can.* Ride a bike and get those pedals spinning round at a crazy rate. Or if you can't ride a bike and you don't have a trike, walk ridiculously quickly, as though playing a childish game. It will give you a buzz, we promise.

Use activity for relaxation by developing your own individual dance routines (see below). Take up swimming with a friend so that you both keep going. Join the local gym and go round the circuit of exercise machines with the encouragement of their staff. Go for long brisk walks, exploring your local parks and footpaths. It doesn't matter what you do – so long as you do more of it. Aim to be up in the activity group above within two months.
Refer to Sections 5, 6 and 7, below.

Under 20: Very inactive
At this level of activity, you are probably sick, disabled, depressed or stuck in someone else's fantasy. If you are none of these things, you badly need to change your priorities and your way of life, because your inactivity is very likely to endanger your health.

Whatever your present state, you can improve it. Do not lose heart. You will be familiar with the saying, the longest journey starts with the first step; it is more than a cliché: it is a truism. Take that step, then the one after; each one after that will be easier. Focus your mind on the goal of a slim and healthy self; do not be distracted by despair at what you think you are now. Concentrate on developing your potential.

If you suffer from illness which makes activity difficult, the chances are that careful activity will actually help your recovery. In our book, *Alternatives to Drugs*, we give specific advice on dealing with illness and disability which you may find useful.

Walking is the best activity to start with for everyone who has use of their legs. Get a pair of good trainers and start to walk, going further and faster every day as you grow fitter. Walk every day, preferably during daylight hours when the sun's light will improve your mental and physical state. If you were to do nothing apart from increase your walking, you would start to shift that fat. But of course, as walking makes you fitter, you will find it easier to move on to more vigorous and varied forms of activity – you will be on a beneficial cycle instead of a dangerous decline.

Refer to Sections 6, 9 and 10, below.

Specific suggestions

Before following any of these suggestions make sure you have completed *both* questionnaires and noted all the sections which are relevant to you.

1) PLATEAUX
When you have reached a certain level of activity and fitness your body adapts to that activity and you settle on a stable plateau. Your regular activity becomes absorbed into your normal routine, and further benefit becomes elusive.

To avoid this you have to change the type and rate of

activity. This keeps your systems guessing and makes them work. If you have been doing basic movements, try using weights to increase the work rate. If you have been mainly walking, try the RCAF fitness routine (Section 4, below). If you run regularly try swimming or bike riding. The objective is to develop the widest possible range of capacity and ability – to become a complete physical person. Move into other areas; do things that emphasise one of the three S's – strength, stamina or suppleness – the one that is your *weakest* area!

Do not become obsessive about time, place or activity. Change enriches life.

2) FASTER = LIGHTER

Whatever movement or activity you are doing, remember that the faster you move the more energy you burn. In crude terms faster equals lighter. So you may need to speed up what you are doing to get more benefit. This has implications other than the simply physical; to sustain faster movement you will need to produce a different hormone mix, and this will help your body refine its shape; you also need to concentrate harder on the precise movement and its energy demands. This improved mental connection will produce high levels of confidence in your ability.

If you want to increase the size of any body area, exercise the muscle group involved with a low number of movements against high resistance, in a gym with weights. If you want to decrease the size of any muscle group use high repetitions against low resistance. Your gym instructor will help you with this sort of specialised body structuring.

3) RUNNING

Running is the most complete form of natural activity. It affects every major body system, and can take each to its limit. Regular running can extend those limits and refine body systems to a very high degree. It is very beneficial for the cardiovascular system, improving circulation and lowering blood pressure; it also improves liver function and capacity; it can change brain chemistry and lift depression, alleviate pain, reduce pre-menstrual tension and period problems. It sheds fat and helps maintain a perfect skin. We admit it, we are hooked. A regular, but varied, running session is highly enjoyable!

How much, or how little, should you run? If you are just beginning, getting on in years or heavy, doing too little is better than doing too much. For the first few outings, do about half of what you believe you could do. See what effects this has on you; if you are stiff, bruised or strained, so that movement is difficult next day – you have overdone it. Wait until you have recovered before trying (less) again.

Remember what you are trying to achieve. Your first stage is to build up enough capacity to enable you to work all those body systems. Take your time on this, it can take a year or two of steady progress, but you will be improving your figure and your health all the time. The second stage is to be able to do enough strenuous activity to persuade your liver to turn on and discharge its glycogen stores. Once this happens you will experience the phenomenon of 'second wind'. On the brink of apparent exhaustion, your liver turns on, and suddenly energy flows freely, you become light and feel you can run for ever. Don't – 20 to 30 minutes will be fine! Finish with a gradual wind down so that you are just jogging when you get home.

As you become more fit it may take more effort to achieve this effect. You may find you have to run further or faster. Either way you should vary your speed and stride length when running. Do not settle down into a mindless pointless jog – running is a dynamic activity that should involve every fibre of your being.

4) RCAF PHYSICAL FITNESS ROUTINE

The advantage of this tried and tested system is that it is comprehensive, and graduated. Buy the book *Physical Fitness* published by Penguin, which explains the whole system. Whatever your state and ability you can follow this routine and gain immediate benefits. It is not geared to fat loss as such; the objective is fitness, but it will get you fit enough to burn that fat.

We use these routines when travelling, when time is short but we want to maintain our state of fitness, and also as a warm-up routine before other activities. You could do the same.

5) TRAIN – NOT STRAIN

Pain is a message of distress. If you experience any pain when exercising, stop. When you have interpreted the message, you can decide whether to go on or not. Minor muscular aches or fatigue that lifts after a short break can be ignored, but not persistent sharp pain. Joint pain should be listened to, as should pain from the chest or respiratory system. Run your activity gently down, keep the affected part loose and mobile, and try again another day.

Do not join those fools who think a pot of gold lies behind the pain barrier. Your objective is to train yourself, to build up capacity and improve ability, not to destroy yourself. Take your time and concentrate on pleasure and enjoyment.

Having said that, there is one exception. Those fit enough to run regularly may notice an occasional twinge in the right side of the chest. This can be the liver saying it does not want to perform today. Try persuasion, but if it is dealing with alcohol from the night before, fighting an infection or otherwise overloaded, it might be wise to listen to it and trot off home.

6) WALKING

We advise everyone to walk briskly – in excess of four miles an hour – for half an hour every day.

For many, this single change in routine will produce a large improvement. When you do it is not important. You might be able to walk to and from work, or part of the journey, or spend half your lunch break walking, or you could make it an evening event.

Whenever you walk, wear comfortable flat shoes. Good quality trainers, those intended for use not fashion, are excellent. For rough or wet ground get traditional stout shoes.

If you have not walked much recently start off with a brisk quarter of an hour and gradually build up. Do not count stop-start shopping, you must walk continuously. When you can cover two miles in around twenty-five minutes, you are probably ready to start doing a little running on your outings! Go on, you can do it!

7) RAISING METABOLISM

The aim of activity is to raise your metabolic rate. Dieting and traditional slimming has the effect of depressing the metabolic rate, which is why dieters tend to get fat. Changing your eating pattern to that described in Chapter 12 will help lift this depression; activity will help it take off.

Without an increase in metabolic rate you will not be able to metabolise fat. It is as simple as that. So increasing activity is essential.

Whatever your current activity level or ability, you can improve it. Understanding why you need to do so should provide enough motivation.

8) TIME FOR SELF

You must be selfish for your own good. You need time and space to achieve your objectives, so make it or take it. And use it to get in touch with yourself.

Try this method. Shut yourself in a room alone; create a soft and warm ambiance. Put on some favourite music that will help you relax. Close your eyes and drift with the music; move with it as you feel; try to get in touch with your innermost feelings. Let them bubble through and surface. Move with the music, stretching, bending, jumping, dancing, rocking, whatever feels good. Gradually build up the speed and intensity of your movements, working through those suppressed feelings as you work muscles and move limbs. When you have gone as far as you can, relax. Shake out your arms and legs, jog on the spot, wind down emotionally, and relax in a warm bath.

It might help to write down anything that struck you as particularly important to your life, your situation or your desires. Having fixed it, you can start to resolve it.

9) MOBILITY

Very few people are totally immobile. The thing to do is to start from where you are and make steady progress to extend your capacity.

Start by moving every joint you can through its full range of movement. Start with your fingers; spread them wide and back, then slowly clench them into a tight fist, repeat as often as you can or like. Then with a loose fist, move your wrist back and forth, up and down, round and round, stretching for the maximum movement. Next the elbow . . . and so on, using every joint to its maximum. Take your time, do movements at odd times. Try it to music.

10) START UP

Why not try dancing? Anyone, even if confined to bed, can undertake some form of enjoyable rhythmic movement to music. Dancing is one of the oldest forms of human recreation (re-creation). It gives us self-expression, relaxation, stimulation and exhilaration; it can provide transcendence, communication and emotional satisfaction. Do not believe you are too old, too big, too awkward or too anything else. None of that is important, forget it. You may be self-conscious, but that can be turned into something valuable by dance – consciousness of self!

Dance can be used to regenerate and extend the very core of your being. Because it is a self-directed activity it will involve many levels of your being, both physical and mental. It will create feedback loops which can build up sensations and energy that can become intense and exhilarating. At other times dance can be a gentle exploration of parts of yourself and your emotions. Whatever, dance will help you unlock and grow.

Activity and tension must be balanced by relaxation. You will find that increased activity will help you to relax more easily, but you may have to work specifically on relaxing to achieve a satisfactory balance in your life.

Make sure that activity is rewarded. You should work on developing a pleasurable relaxation routine with as much effort as you work on activity. It might include a warm bath, a sensuous shower or massage by a friend or partner. This will increase your self-value and fulfilment and is just as necessary to you.

Yoga and meditation are good formal methods which you might consider. Otherwise anything which helps you unwind when you need to should be explored. If there is a significant block, say with a relationship, you must face the cause and try to resolve it. Having your own time and space might be the enabling factor you need.

Exertion breaks down muscle fibres, depletes energy stores and fires up the metabolism. All this generates debris that has to be cleared, and demands for renewal and re-stocking which have to be met.

Most of this happens when you are asleep. There is a basic switch in the brain; when we are awake and active it is set to use and go, when we are asleep it is set to recoup and repair. It is during this time that our metabolism will be shifting fat, reshaping our muscles, increasing its own capacity for future demands and re-charging liver and muscle glycogen stores.

If you go short of sleep you will disrupt this essential work. You must do whatever is necessary to ensure a good night's sleep every night.

You don't lose weight only while you are awake!

Whatever your current state it is important to start from

where you are. Ideally we should maintain a balanced mixture of mental and physical activity in our lives. We should have skills in both spheres which would enhance our options for expression and satisfaction. Unfortunately, life tends to push us behind desks, into mindless repetitive tasks, into the roles others design for us, or it leaves us isolated with a minimal role or function.

In this context exercise and other activities designed to have specific effects can be seen in two ways: first as the substitutes for an unsatisfactory reality that they undeniably are, but secondly, as a way of significantly changing that reality for the better. Exercise not only improves you, it will also help create a better reality. Every demand you make for physical expression makes the next one easier; the more we make this demand the more it will become a normal part of a more satisfactory life.

When you have started on a course of activities, repeat the questionnaires at monthly intervals, to check progress and make sure you are moving on to areas that match your new ability.

CHAPTER 14

Mind and Metabolism

You know what you should eat tó be slim and stay that way. You know that activity burns off fat. Yet you are unable to make this knowledge work for you. You try to sustain the willpower that should bring success, yet your resolve breaks down time and again.

Do you recognise yourself? If so, your problem starts in your mind: your emotional, irrational self is controlling your behaviour, in conflict with your thinking self. To make matters worse, that errant child-self is likely to be working in tandem with the parts of your brain that control your metabolic processes and your hormones.

Conflict between what we *think* we want and what the powerful emotional levels of our selves permit is very common. All of us suffer from this kind of problem to some degree, doing things that we intended not to do, breaking sensible rules that we set ourselves, failing to meet our own standards for reasons that we do not completely under-stand. Of course, we vary; each individual is a unique mix. Your brother may have no trouble at all with eating – but he cannot resist infidelity. Your friend may be unable to resist gambling. And you sometimes cannot stop yourself eating. Or drinking, if that is what piles on the fat.

You may see your excess weight as a major problem, but in reality it should be the relatively trivial focus for concern that distracts you from a more difficult problem that you have been unable to face. You *think* you do not want the weight but it may be that the emotional self that tells you to eat actually *does* want that weight, and that's where your conflict lies. The questionnaire below will help you to find out.

FAT AS AN ASSET

Because we are trying to uncover motives that are not readily accessible to the conscious mind, we are not looking for rational or unprejudiced answers in this questionnaire. Try to get in touch with your *feelings*. This may be easier if you imagine yourself as a fat person and then as a thin person in situations which are relevant to the questions. If you can imagine yourself coping better when you are fat, you have touched on a motive for staying that way.

(Note the degree of agreement between your feelings and the statement by scoring 5 if you definitely agree; 4 if you agree somewhat; 3 if your feelings are neutral; 2 if you disagree somewhat; and 1 if you absolutely disagree.)

1. I feel stronger when I am bigger; a big person is a force to be reckoned with.
2. It would be hard to cope with the sexual advances that I would attract if I were slim.
3. Slim people are not cuddly.
4. It's useful to be big because you get noticed, and not just as a sex object.
5. Fat is a protective layer – I hide behind it.
6. Slim people are cold and mean.

Add your scores to give a total figure for the Fat as an Asset scale.

Over 22

Your fat has definite positive value for you. You have to decide whether you really do want to lose it or whether slimness would be so uncomfortable for you that the potential disadvantages outweigh the advantages. To continue trying to fight the flab when you have such strong motives for retaining it will be difficult.

There are two ways of resolving this conflict. One is to be fat, accept it, and understand how it makes sense to you. The other is to work through your unconscious motivation, bring it up into your consciousness and acknowledge that you are investing power and strength in your fat that you could integrate into your picture of your inner, slim self. By making warmth, strength and other positive qualities into aspects of fatness, you are denying their reality as facets of your own personality. Read Susie Orbach's *Fat is a Feminist Issue*. Even if you do not see yourself as a feminist, the book contains valuable insights.

For some people, counselling or psychotherapeutic techniques like rebirthing can produce dramatic results by helping them to understand their reasons for being fat. You may need to reassess the way you think and feel about your parents: your fat could be a focus of rebellion against a mother who wanted you to achieve more than she did; or your dependence on alcohol could be the way you suppress the anger you feel towards your father. When you can live your own life for yourself, you may no longer need to be fat.

You are likely to find that you can settle on less fat while remaining cuddly, warm and comfortable. But probably you do not, and should not, wish to be thin. Just aim for a healthy lifestyle!

11–21

Although you have some interest in being fat, this is unlikely to be sufficient to account for a serious weight problem. But you should be aware that your desire to lose weight is tempered by motives which will tend to undermine your resolve.

Reconsider the target size or weight that you have been trying to achieve. Have you adopted some standard for thinness that is inappropriate for you? Perhaps you are trying to emulate a body type that does not fit in with the way you live your life or the people you live with. If others who are important to you value your plumpness, you would be ill-advised to try to become too lean.

Under 10
For you, fat has very little value. Being fat is an entirely negative experience; you feel that slim people have all the advantages. So because – or *if* – you are fat, you will dislike yourself all the more.

You should consider the possibility that you are setting yourself up for failure. If life for slim people is so good, perhaps you fear having to meet your own expectations of slimness. Perhaps people would *not* find you any more attractive if you were slim. Perhaps your problems go deeper than that, and the failures that you attribute to the fat would have occurred even if you had been slim. Dare you find out? Sometimes it is easier to fail at the first hurdle than risk failure at one that seems more important. You can avoid the test of slimness by staying fat.

Of course, such logic as this – which is characteristic of the less rational but often more powerful parts of our minds – does not actually benefit us. Fear of failure leads to failure. So look closely at your attitudes to yourself and the importance you put on slimness. Do not hold back from accomplishing what you want to do because you think you are not slim enough; and never use your size as an excuse that allows you to avoid accepting responsibility for your life.

Eating problems are part of a larger picture of unhappiness which usually goes right back to childhood. They grow in importance and become harder to deal with when we are anxious, angry, frustrated or unhappy. At such times, not only do many people turn to the chocolates or empty the fridge, but their bodies seem to react particularly badly to the food loaded in under these circumstances. A feast eaten joyfully turns to fat much less readily than food stuffed miserably in an attempt to feed the hungry heart. (The hormones which are linked with alertness, activity and happiness are also those which release fat from storage – adrenalin and nor-adrenalin. When levels of these hormones are high, you are less likely to gain weight.)

Yet misery and guilt are characteristic of the compulsive eater who falls from the virtuous diet and binges on forbidden foods. She eats alone as the tears spill from her eyes, cursing herself yet unable to stop. She eats until her belly feels sore and bloated and the cupboards are bare. Some women have killed themselves by overeating this way. It is especially dangerous after a strict diet – but it is also a common reaction to dieting. Particularly if that man still rejects you when you're slim.

Is your weight problem really a symptom of emotional stress? If so, you must concentrate on solving the problems that lie behind it. Try another questionnaire . . .

EMOTIONAL AND SOCIAL PROBLEMS
(Mark your degree of agreement with each statement by underlining the answer that best fits your feelings.)

1. The slightest upset makes me cry; I am on the edge of tears most of the time.
   Agree absolutely; agree somewhat; neutral; disagree somewhat; disagree absolutely.

2. I often feel empty inside.
   Agree absolutely; agree somewhat; neutral; disagree somewhat; disagree absolutely.

3. I enjoy my life.
   Agree absolutely; agree somewhat; neutral; disagree somewhat; disagree absolutely.

4. I feel that I am not in control of my own life.
   Agree absolutely; agree somewhat; neutral; disagree somewhat; disagree absolutely.

5. I am hardly ever bored or lonely.
   Agree absolutely; agree somewhat; neutral; disagree somewhat; disagree absolutely.

6. I cannot cope with the demands made on me.
   Agree absolutely; agree somewhat; neutral; disagree somewhat; disagree absolutely.

7. I wish I could have been a child for ever.
   Agree absolutely; agree somewhat; neutral; disagree somewhat; disagree absolutely.

8. When I was a child, my mother seemed very happy.
   Agree absolutely; agree somewhat; neutral; disagree somewhat; disagree absolutely.

9. I sleep easily and deeply.
   Agree absolutely; agree somewhat; neutral; disagree somewhat; disagree absolutely.

10. Other people prevent me from achieving what I want.
    Agree absolutely; agree somewhat; neutral; disagree somewhat; disagree absolutely.

11. I eat substantially more when I am unhappy.
    Agree absolutely; agree somewhat; neutral; disagree somewhat; disagree absolutely.

12. I have a satisfying sex life.
    Agree absolutely; agree somewhat; neutral; disagree somewhat; disagree absolutely.

Score table

	Agree			Disagree	
	absolutely	somewhat	neutral	somewhat	absolutely
1.	5	4	3	2	1
2.	5	4	3	2	1
3.	1	2	3	4	5
4.	5	4	3	2	1
5.	1	2	3	4	5
6.	5	4	3	2	1
7.	5	4	3	2	1
8.	1	2	3	4	5
9.	1	2	3	4	5
10.	5	4	3	2	1
11.	5	4	3	2	1
12.	1	2	3	4	5

Add together the figures for all the questions to give a total
score for Social/Emotional Problems.

INTERPRETING YOUR EMOTIONAL/SOCIAL PROBLEM SCORE

Over 40

Your emotional state definitely contributes to your weight
problem. It does this in a number of ways: it can cause you
to eat to numb your feelings; it can depress your whole
system so that you can't use the energy that comes from
burning food, which gets stored as fat instead; and if you
are taking tablets to help you cope with your unhappiness,
they can also make you put on weight.

You will probably lose weight quite effortlessly when you
are feeling happier; you will certainly find it much easier to
shed that unwanted fat. So do not despair. Do not use your
guilt about being fat as another way of chastising yourself;
you are fat because you are unhappy, not unhappy because
you are fat. The fat is a symptom, nothing else.

You will be glad to know that the action you should take

to get your body to burn fat faster will help to solve your emotional problems. Impossible? Far from it. Among the natural remedies for anxiety and depression are eating a balanced diet and increasing your activity level. Read Chapters 12 and 13 and act on them. These actions will ensure that the biochemical balance in your body and brain is conducive to happiness, while inactivity and a poor diet will make you more susceptible to emotional illness. Spend more time outdoors during daylight hours; whether you walk the dog, tend your vegetable garden or sit in the park matters less than just being out there in natural light with other growing, living things.

You may blame fat for your unhappiness because you cannot face the possibility that something you value highly is the source of your internal conflict. Depression is most often associated with marital problems or difficulties in relationships with the people who are most important to you. If you feel you cannot resolve these difficulties, getting fat and attributing your problems to that allows you to avoid confronting what seems like an insoluble problem. It is no solution, of course; but you may need help in finding a more effective answer. Counselling could help you see a way through. The number of your local marriage guidance council (now renamed Relate) will be in the telephone directory; their trained counsellors can help resolve any relationship problems, whether they concern a partner or not.

There are many other steps you can take to recover from your emotional problems but this is not the place to deal with them in the detail that you may require. We give more information in our book *Alternatives to Drugs*.

20–40
Emotional difficulties are relevant to your weight problem. Your state (and your weight) will fluctuate from time to time, as your emotional state changes. Read the advice

above and concentrate on *dealing* with things that are making you unhappy.

Under 20
You are emotionally well-balanced – at least, at the moment! Your weight problems are not likely to be due to unhappiness.

LEARNING TO COPE WITH COMPULSIVE EATING
Even if you have sorted out your most pressing problems, you cannot expect to be totally stable and sensible all the time. Everyone is subject to mood swings, and if you have learnt to respond to downswings by overeating, you could find that you continue to have recurring weight problems even if you know perfectly well how to maintain yourself at a sensible size. So how do you stop yourself turning to food when your body doesn't need it?

The first step is to ensure that your body indeed does not need it. Many people only begin to suffer from severe bouts of compulsive eating after they start dieting. It is a reaction to deprivation and over-control; once control starts to go, once you lose that feeling of strength that keeps the conscious mind on top, the desperation that you stifled throughout the dieting weeks boils up with uncontrolled power.

If you are actually on a diet when you slip like this, the diet mentality will push you further down the slope. It is likely to initiate a pattern of wild swings of eating and fat. When your desire for forbidden food overcomes your will, you feel awful because you have broken the rules of the diet. You have failed, you are a failure, you might as well give up on yourself, you are hateful anyway, you might just as well eat . . .

Freeing yourself from the diet mentality defuses the whole situation. Eating a packet (or two) of biscuits is no longer wicked: it's just irrational. It's human. We are all irrational at times. Let it happen. It doesn't make you into a monster and its effects will not be so terrible. So what? You can eat if you want to! Slim people do not worry about the weight they may put on with a blow-out – it will come off again as easily as it went on. Remember, if you are to stop being a fat person, you must stop thinking like one. Adopt the optimistic slim perspective.

Dieting is a process which depends on internal conflict. It relies on your ability to suppress your internal knowledge of what, and how much, you want to eat. To be free of weight problems, you have to try to get back to a pre-diet innocence, when you were able to respond not to what you thought you *should* do, but to what you *wanted* to do. How easily you can achieve this depends on your personality and your early experiences; if your family made you feel guilty for refusing food and pressed you always to finish what was put on your plate, you may find there are emotional blocks on your perception of hunger and satiation which you must overcome.

Freeing yourself from the diet guilt allows you to get to know yourself and to enjoy your occasional bouts of gluttony. Spoil yourself! You need spoiling sometimes. We all do. Enjoy your food. When you stop enjoying it, you will be able to stop eating. You are going to eat: so make the most of it. Acknowledge that *you* have made the choice. This integrates the different levels of your being, to give you an internal balance that is conducive to both emotional and physical health.

When you feel the desire for a binge coming on, think about what you really want to eat. The guilt reaction you used to have probably never allowed you to experience your desire fully so that you could indulge yourself properly. Many binges start with foods that are thoroughly unappealing – stale crusts, yukky leftovers, stuff that you would never consider giving to anyone else to eat. You give it to yourself as a mark of your low self-esteem. So cut that nonsense! Feeling bad about yourself will do you no good at all.

Mentally test different foods against your appetite. What would you really like to eat? What would make your whole system feel best? If the answer is 'a chocolate éclair', then go and get a chocolate éclair. Eat it slowly, savouring every morsel. Do not allow the slightest twinge of guilt to enter your consciousness. You are solving your chocolate éclair problem, and it is good for you to do so. Maybe you want a second one to satisfy your desire. Get another. Eat it slowly, with full awareness that you have tuned into a personal appetite and you are satisfying it.

You may want chocolate éclairs for a week – but by the end of that week you will know that you do not want chocolate éclairs at all, that they do not actually make you feel good any more. You will be more in tune with yourself, less controlled by outside rules. Those outside rules and your assumptions about eating contributed to your weight problem. Now, you are able to make your own decisions.

When you feel guilty about eating, you eat with minimal awareness. The pleasure that you crave is lost. Enjoying your food, and enjoying the sensation of satisfying appetite, will help you to use food as it should be used – for your benefit. Becoming more aware of the real effects of different foods eaten without guilt or anxiety will help you to adopt eating habits that match your needs. This is the way healthy slim people behave. It is a crucial step towards lifetime slenderness.

There is an important difference between eating wisely because it makes you feel good and controlling your eating to avoid being fat. Positive motivation involves acceptance of yourself and your appetites and provides a sound basis for long-term success.

Controlling your eating with rigid rules and willpower has the opposite effect. It creates the potential for disaster. Disaster for you may have been compulsive eating and fat; but even if your control is so strong that you are able to get slim and stay that way, your obsession would merely bring disaster in another shape.

Anorexia nervosa represents the ultimate triumph of the will over appetite. It has a subtle addictive attraction for people who lack belief in their own competence yet set themselves the highest standards. By refusing to give in to the desire to eat, anorexics prove that they are strong, they are in control; every day the anorexic starves, proves her toughness. While she starves she can be proud of herself. Yet underneath, her desperate lack of confidence is reflected in the rejection of a mature fleshy body.

Anorexia is a very dangerous condition and difficult to get out of. The voluntary control with which it starts can change to involuntary starvation when the victim's body and mind come to reject nourishment totally.

Anorexia's close cousin is bulimia. Nobody knows how many slender adolescents keep their waif-like looks by vomiting secretly after every meal: it is not something that can be discussed in polite society. The shame that surrounds bulimia adds to the burden of self-rejection that leads to its development in the first place.

Compulsive eating, bulimia and anorexia are all part of the same pattern: a pattern that has developed because the society we have created puts terrible pressure on many people by failing to acknowledge their real needs. Our cultural attitudes to fat, dieting and eating have created conditions that are making increasing numbers of people mentally and physically ill.

CHAPTER 15

Weight? No Problem!

In Chapter 1 we promised that you would be well on the road to successfully controlling your weight, fat and body shape when you had read this book. If you have done the questionnaires, answered the questions honestly and followed our recommendations, weight will no longer be a problem. Any excess fat will be disappearing as your physical state improves; soon you could be feeling stronger, fitter, and leaner than you have for a long time. Understanding the nature of the problem you had and seeing your way forward will be enough to set the necessary changes in motion.

When you have accepted that understanding, you will have learnt to accept yourself in a way that never seemed possible when weight was a problem. Those who try to conquer their weight by depriving and punishing themselves, dividing the controlling mind from the unruly body, fail because the body evades the trickery of the calorie count and counter-attacks with redoubled efficiency. Such simplistic mechanistic answers create more problems than they solve.

Once you think like a slim person, you stop arbitrarily depriving yourself of nourishment as dieters do. Instead, you act like a slim person and your body responds by shedding the fat that it no longer needs. With body and mind working in harmony, long-term success comes within reach.

You are no longer the victim of cultural assumptions about fat and dieting. Dieters' trust in others – whether parents, the food and chemical industries, journalists or diet doctors – leads them to damage themselves in their perpetual war with weight. But you now know that the answer lies in trusting yourself, respecting your body's needs and the way you function, and trusting internal cues. You will have gained a large degree of control over your life and the particular factors that conspired to make you fat. And you will be equipped to deal with them.

Once you have worked through your initial programme, go back and answer the questionnaires again. You will have changed, and so will your answers. You will find that you are directed towards actions which will help you to achieve your ultimate goal: a lifestyle that allows you to get on with living and forget fat and weight.

In this final chapter we will return to some of the themes which appeared earlier in the book, to give you a broader vision of things which obsess old-fashioned dieters. We hope this will help you to see them in perspective so that you can judge their real importance.

The first point is the question of weight loss. Throughout this book we have used the words 'weight' and 'fat' as if they were more or less interchangeable. But, depending on the way you act, you can lose fat while gaining weight, or lose weight but not fat.

This presents a problem because weight is not the important issue. Unfortunately, factors that do matter, such as the proportion and distribution of fat on your body and the way it affects you as an individual, are very difficult to measure. Factors that are easy to measure, such as calories and weight, tend to get picked out and endowed with characteristics which, although actually irrelevant to our interests, are given exaggerated importance. Thus somebody, somewhere, devises a table of height (also conveniently easy to measure) and weight, and makes arbitrary decisions about what is normal, over- or under-weight for any given height; and because our height is more or less fixed, we worry about weight.

Weight, like most simple measurements, misses the point. You can be a stone 'under-weight' and still be fat and shapeless; similarly, you may be a stone 'over-weight' and breathtakingly beautiful. Crude measurements of weight can be totally misleading.

To distinguish between fat and weight, you have to learn to trust your eyes and develop your judgement. As a first step, throw away your bathroom scales. Get yourself a full-length mirror and put it in the bathroom or bedroom where you will see your naked self every day. Transfer your allegiance from figures on the scale to your figure in the flesh. We quoted Judy Mazel's suggestion that you treat your bathroom scales as your lover: what a heartless lover to choose! Now you can get down to a much more real and rewarding relationship. Look in your mirror; there is your lover: you. You must love and respect yourself. Without love for yourself, you will never live happily in your own body and you will never be able to love another person fully.

Accepting yourself includes accepting the reality of what you are and what is possible for you. Your body type may not be the elongated image of the fashion magazines; you have to accept that and not try to achieve an ideal that can never be you. Weight is always a problem for those who insist on aiming at a level below that which is natural for them and their lifestyle.

Your ideal shape and size cannot be judged in relation to the current cultural ideal, only in relation to your real needs. Cultural ideals are fickle; that of one decade is superseded by another the next. Progressively slimmer, more masculine women have been admired recently in western culture; the sad result is that many women, whose lack of self-acceptance undermines their confidence and independence of judgement, reject their feminine shape.

With the cultural ideal distorting your vision, you look at yourself and find your body unattractive by comparison. To make matters worse, many people build up pictures of themselves which magnify their perceived failings. The strength of the cultural ideal in conjunction with lack of acceptance of self creates a distortion of perception which can become extreme. The anorexic, all skin and bone, looks in the mirror and sees herself rippling with fat. You are securely in control when you have a clear and positive view of yourself; but this requires that you adjust the inner picture as well as the outer reality.

You achieve this by allowing yourself to enjoy living within your own body, through active acceptance of your appetites and growing abilities. Using your body in enjoyable activity is an important part of this process. Fighting flab used to be a battle with yourself; now you understand how the total balance of your life determines your body composition, you can win without struggling. Our society and the world at large is doing so much to keep you fat that the last thing you want is conflict with yourself.

Your success demands that you be sufficiently selfish to take the time and space you need, to stretch, pamper, reward and enjoy yourself. It may also be the time to think of others, taking your friends with you, sharing your knowledge and pleasure with them, extending the eating and activity lessons into your family.

The recommendations we have made in this book are not only relevant to becoming slim. They are based firmly on the essential foundations for a healthy life, and so are applicable to everyone. Our books on avoiding heart disease, on being healthy without drugs, on improving immunity to infection, all share the same areas of common concern: nutrition, pollution, activity, self-acceptance. These are areas of life where human needs are not being met, where priorities other than the quality of life determine policies that affect us all. It is difficult to be slim in a world where so many pressures conspire to create fatness; it is difficult to be healthy in a world where health comes second to economics. The quality of your flesh depends on the quality of your life as a whole; narrow concepts, limited aims and simplistic answers are not enough to create the wholesome reality we all need.

Your determination to move towards a healthier way of living will affect those around you. Eventually, the demand for our right to positive health will affect decision-making at all levels. By our active participation we protect not only ourselves but our children, their children, and life to come.

Bibliography

CHAPTERS 1 AND 2

Beller, A. S., *Fat and Thin*. Farrar, Straus & Giroux, 1977

Cannon, G. and Einzig, H., *Dieting Makes You Fat*. Sphere Books, 1984

Forbes, G. B., *Human Body Composition*. Springer-Verlag, 1987

Mazel, J., *The Beverly Hills Diet*. Arrow Books, 1982

Schwartz, B., *Diets Don't Work*. Columbus Books, 1986

Stern, J., 'Diet and Exercise'. In: Greenwood, M.R.C. (ed.), *Obesity*. Churchill Livingstone, 1983

CHAPTER 3

Bland, J., *Medical Applications of Clinical Nutrition*. Keats, 1981

BMA Board of Science: Policy Statement on Very Low Calorie Diets, British Medical Association, 1988

Committee on Medical Aspects of Food Policy, *The Use of Very Low Calorie Diets in Obesity*. Department of Health and Social Security/HMSO, 1987

Doull, J. *et al.* (eds.), *Casarett and Doull's Toxicology, The Basic Science of Poisons*. Macmillan, 1980

Howard, A., *The Cambridge Diet*. Corgi, 1986

Marks, J. and Howard, A., *The Cambridge Diet: A Manual for Practitioners*. MTP Press, 1986

Veitch, A., 'Old Saw Could Save Old Bones'. Guardian, 5 November 1987

'The Very Low Calorie Diet'. Editorial in *The Lancet*, 1 September 1984, p.500

Wadden, T. A., *et al.*, 'Very Low Calorie Diets: their efficacy, safety and future'. *Annals of Internal Medicine*, 99, 1983

Wilson, J. H. P., 'Cardiac complications of drastic weight reduction'. *Netherlands Journal of Medicine*, 29, 1986

CHAPTER 4

AMA Council on Foods and Nutrition, 'A Critique of Low Carbohydrate Ketogenic Weight Reduction Regimens'. *Journal of the American Medical Association*, 224, 1973

Atkins, R., *Dr Atkins' Diet Revolution*. David McKay, 1972

Bland, J., *Medical Applications of Clinical Nutrition*. Keats, 1981

Danbrot, M., *The 4-Day Wonder Diet*. Bantam Books, 1986

Dwyer, J., 'Sixteen popular diets'.

In: A. J. Stunkard (ed.), *Obesity*. W. B. Saunders, 1980

Rudin, D. O., 'Omega-3 Essential Fatty Acids in Medicine'. *1984–5 Yearbook of Nutritional Medicine*

Stillman, I. M. and Baker, S. S., *The Doctor's Quick Weight Loss Diet*. Prentice-Hall, 1967

Taller, H., *Calories Don't Count*. Corgi, 1963

Tarnower, H. And Baker, S. S., *The Complete Scarsdale Medical Diet*. Bantam Books, 1985

Taylor, R., *My Life on a Diet*. G. P. Putnam's Sons, 1986

CHAPTER 5

Bruch, H., *Eating Disorders: Obesity, Anorexia Nervosa and the Person Within*. Routledge & Kegan Paul, 1974

Mazel, J., *The Beverly Hills Diet*. Arrow Books, 1982

Passwater, R. A. and Cranton, E. M., *Trace Elements, Hair Analysis and Nutrition*. Keats, 1983

Stern, J., 'Diet and Exercise'. In: Greenwood, M.R.C. (ed.), *Obesity*. Churchill Livingstone, 1983

CHAPTER 6

Barker, L. M., *The Psychobiology of Human Food Selection*. Avi, 1982

Davies, S. and Stewart, A., *Nutritional Medicine*. Pan Books, 1987

Eyton, A., *The F-Plan*. Penguin, 1982

CHAPTER 7

Barker, L. M., *The Psychobiology of Human Food Selection*. Avi, 1982

Forbes, G. B., *Human Body Composition*. Springer-Verlag, 1987

Katahn, M., *The Rotation Diet*. Bantam Books, 1988

Katahn, M., *The 200 Calorie Solution*. Norton, 1984

Weight Watchers Quick Start Plus Programme. Weight Watchers International, Inc.

CHAPTER 8

Diamond, H. & M., *Fit for Life*. Bantam, 1987

Forbes, A., *The Bristol Diet*. Century, 1984

Grant, D. and Joice, J., *Food Combining for Health*. Thorsons, 1984

Irvine, L., *Castaway*. Gollancz, 1983

Kenton, L., *The Biogenic Diet*. Arrow, 1986

CHAPTER 11

Hanssen, M., *E for Additives*. Thorsons, 1984

Johnson, C. and Melville, A., *Hay Fever: No Need to Suffer*. Corgi, 1984

Melville, A. and Johnson, C., *Persistent Fat and How to Lose It*. Century, 1986

Melville, A. and Johnson, C., *Alternatives to Drugs*. Fontana, 1987

Royal Canadian Air Force, *Physical Fitness*. Penguin, 1964

CHAPTER 12

Gear, A., *The New Organic Food Guide*. J. M. Dent & Sons, 1987

Trowell, H. C. and Burkitt, D. P. (eds.), *Western Diseases: Their Emergence and Prevention*. Edward Arnold, 1981

Walker, C. and Cannon, G., *The Food Scandal*. Century, 1984

Yudkin, J., *Pure, White and Deadly*. Davis-Poynter, 1972

CHAPTER 13

Brooks, G. A. and Fahey, T. D., *Exercise physiology: Human Bionergetics and its Applications*. Wiley, 1984

Mutrie, N., 'The psychological effects of exercise for women'. In: Macleod, D. *et al.*, *Exercise: Benefits, Limits and Adaptations*. E & F. N. Spon, 1987

Prior, J. C., 'Exercise-related adaptive changes of the menstrual cycle'. In: Macleod, D. *et al.*, *Exercise: Benefits, Limits and Adaptations*. E & F. N. Spon, 1987

CHAPTER 14

Bruch, H., *Eating Disorders: Obesity, Anorexia Nervosa and the Person Within*. Routledge & Kegan Paul, 1974

Orbach, S., *Fat is a Feminist Issue*. Hamlyn Paperbacks, 1979

Roth, G., *Feeding the Hungry Heart: The Experience of Compulsive Eating*. Grafton Books, 1986

Index